HOLY PEOPLE, HOLY LIVES

HOLY
People
HOLY
Lives

Law and Gospel in **BIOETHICS**

Richard C. Eyer

SAINT LOUIS

To my wife
With a grateful heart for years of support ...

Copyright © 2000 Richard C. Eyer
Published by Concordia Publishing House
3558 S. Jefferson Avenue, St. Louis, MO 63118-3968
Manufactured in the United States of America

Library of Congress Cataloging-in-Publication Data

Eyer, Richard C., 1939-
    Holy people, holy lives : law and Gospel in bioethics / Richard C. Eyer.
        p. cm.
Includes bibliographical references.
    ISBN 0-570-05255-6
    1. Medical ethics. 2. Bioethics. 3. Christian ethics. I. Title.
    R725.56 .E94 2000
    174'.2—dc21   00-008495

1 2 3 4 5 6 7 8 9 10   09 08 07 06 05 04 03 02 01 00

Contents

Introduction

This is a book about *ethics*. Not many people will pick up a book on this subject but if I tell you, for example, that classical ethics is about being a good, moral person I hope I might tempt you to read further. I might also pique your interest by telling you that this is a *practical* book intended to help you make moral choices faithful to your calling as a Christian. So this is a book for Christians first of all, but also a book for anyone else wishing to learn more about the biblical message and ethics.

More specifically, this is a book about *bioethics*. Whereas ethics might be understood to be about the morality of how we ought to live together, bioethics deals with the ethics of making choices available to us as a result of breakthroughs in medical technology: genetic engineering (altering of genes), in vitro fertilization (creating a human embryo in the laboratory), artificial insemination (with or without the use of donor sperm or egg), surrogate motherhood (carrying someone else's child in utero for nine months), cloning (reproduction without sex), abortion (the killing of a fetus), infanticide (the killing of newborns), the withholding or withdrawal of treatment in illness, physician-assisted suicide, and euthanasia. Choices in all these areas have become available to us and yet we are often unaware of the meanings or implications of these choices for our life together as a society and for our relationship with God.

Christians have always turned to the Bible as the source for evaluating our relationship with God and how we are to live. Some have pointed out that the Bible doesn't address issues stemming from opportunities provided by new technologies. Yet the Bible does talk about the meanings of our life together in relationship to God. Indeed, the Word of God addresses what it means for us both to bear the image of God while at the same time being corrupted by our sinful human nature.

Human nature is skewed toward self-interest in this fallen world. We do not naturally seek God. In times of suffering we grasp for control of our lives rather than entrust them to God in the face of our own weakness and helplessness. We attempt to take charge of our own destiny rather than wait patiently for the will of God to unfold. In so doing, we reject the one in whose image we are made, asserting our own autonomy instead. The Bible declares that the victory of Jesus' death on the cross overcomes all this resistance and gives new life to those who learn to fear, love, and trust in God. From the perspective of this new life in Christ we come to see things in a new light much more so than we did when *self* was the measure of all things. This new perspective has implications for every area of life, including bioethics.

Whether you are looking for general ethical guidelines or for answers to questions in the area of bioethics, I must warn you that I am not writing a "how-to" manual with specific instructions or rules to follow in determining right from wrong. Surely God has set limits beyond which we may not go, but the Christian ethic is more than knowing our limits. It is about the new life created by the Gospel of Jesus Christ that gives meaning to all that we are and do. And it is my aim to present the Gospel as the grace of God that shapes our ethic as Christians.

What I have to say carries with it more than thirty years background in ministry as parish pastor, hospital chaplain, and, most recently, college professor. The Bible is God's Word to us about reality, describing the way things are in this world and what God has done about them. This Word of God is the foundation for the Christian's ethic.

The Bible is not first and foremost about ethics. It is first of all about God's promise and fulfillment in sending His Son, Jesus Christ our Lord, to redeem the world and to set it right again. The Gospel is the good news of the transformation of reality God has brought about through His Son that we "may be His own and live under Him in His kingdom, and serve Him in everlasting righteousness, innocence and blessedness." The biblical message is not so much about what we must ethically do for God as it is about what God has done for us in Jesus Christ. It is Jesus' death and resurrection that has made us holy and that enables us to live holy lives by the power of the Holy Spirit at work in us. I will attempt to develop this truth and its implications as it relates to us in the issues of bioethics today.

1

Making Ethical Decisions

A critical-care physician meets with the family of a patient in the intensive care lounge and tells them that their mother is critically ill and that even if she survives she will probably be left with some brain damage. The physician must make decisions and the family is asked for their wishes to be made known. The decisions have to do ultimately with determining whether the patient is to be provided with what the physician calls "life support" or whether the patient is "allowed to die."

What is the family to say? After minimally absorbing the initial shock of the situation and without having much time to resolve the emotional impact of such news, someone in the family usually makes the comment, "She wouldn't want to live that way," meaning that she herself would choose death rather than live this way. This family member might well be right in his assessment of her wishes. Decision-making today is heavily weighted on the side of honoring the patient's right to self-determination.

It is important to observe at this point that there has been no conversation between doctor and family or between family members themselves about the ethics or morality of the decision this family is being asked to make. Considerations entering the decision-making process are practical, not ethical in the classical sense of that word. And there is little, if any, spiritual concern for the intentions of God in how we live life in allegiance to Him. Even if the family does share a faith in God, the connections between the will of God and this situation may seem vague and confusing, involving us in ambiguities we would rather not face.

The family therefore resorts to the practical approach of problem solving. They make a decision based on the outcome they want for their mother (and perhaps themselves) and not necessarily on the ethical implications of their decision in relationship to God. Indeed, they may not even know there are any such implications. The practical nature of this conversation between doctor and family leads us to believe that if the patient cannot be restored to reasonable health, it would be better for her not to live. On the basis of this practicality the decision will be made to withdraw support in order, as the physician said, "to allow death."

The ethical question they have not faced, however, is whether they are in reality "allowing" her to die rather than intentionally causing death. The truth is that nothing in the conversation has indicated that she is, in fact, dying. The only question that has been raised is about the quality of life, and this is an uncertain basis on which to make an ethical decision.

We should observe some important things about this approach to decision-making in medical ethics today.[1] First, we ought to be aware that ethics today is not what it used to be. Ethics today is not about choosing between what is morally right and wrong. And even if the decision of right and wrong is applicable in some circumstances, ethics is no longer about choosing between them on the basis of an objective moral standard. A discussion about morality is always subjective, relying on each person to determine what is moral for himself or herself only. As we shall see, the separation of ethics from objective moral standards began some generations ago. Today, when hospital medical ethics committees discuss a case, they do not evaluate the moral integrity of their options. They review whether or not proper procedures have been followed that are both legal and in compliance with accepted medical protocol.

Since about the middle of the twentieth century, medical ethics has been reduced to the measure of its *utilitarian* and *emotive* value, according to whether the options are *practically* and *emotionally* satisfying. As in the case of this family, the concern is for practical outcome: "What will we do with mother if she can't care for herself? Will she be a burden to herself and to others?" The way the question is posed almost seems to dictate the answer when practicality becomes the norm for problem solving. Of course, in a sense these practical questions are important for they identify real problems to be faced, but practical questions are not the first questions that need to be asked. Emotional concerns for the patient and family also need our attention, but moral questions, rather than practical ones, are of first importance in determining one's integrity and faithfulness to God.

Those who are concerned with moral integrity without appropriate attention to practical problems risk being accused of caring more about right and wrong than about the patient. There is a grain of truth in this, but only a grain. Jesus Himself criticized the Pharisees for being more concerned with the Law than with people. Nor is it appropriate for us to avoid the physical and emotional needs of people in crisis, lest we be accused of insensitivity. Righteous indignation, even for the best of reasons, always presents us with the danger of forgetting the persons involved in the dilemma.

Yet to be concerned primarily with practicality and emotional needs leads us into naïvete and sentimentality. Practicality can arise out of naïvete, because it addresses only the immediate needs and does not care about the long-range consequences for people. Instant gratification is a way of life in our culture. Meeting emotional needs can turn to sentimentality when feelings lead to self-pity and self-indulgence. But for purposes of objectivity and a critical examination of bioethics and its issues, we need to go beyond concerns of practicality and emotional satisfaction.

Before we can know what to do and how to respond we must look at the meaning of issues facing us. This book is not intended, therefore, as a book on practical solutions to ethical dilemmas. It is, rather, a book about how to live faithfully in response to the Gospel of Jesus Christ.[2]

THE PERSONAL ETHIC

In the case presented at the beginning of this chapter it is apparent that, although the conversation about what to do with the patient gives little evidence of an outward show of emotion, the decision-making is nevertheless emotionally laden and burdensome. We cannot but identify ourselves with the patient or family, and we see ourselves in that situation, a situation no human being would choose to be in, yet one we may all face someday. In making an ethical decision, it would not be surprising to find ourselves scrambling to find ways to overcome the loss of control and helplessness we feel. Such an urgent crisis causes great discomfort, to say the least. Decision-making is heavily influenced by feelings of helplessness, fear, guilt, even anger and resentment at having to make such a decision.

In the contemporary approach to ethics, the value placed on resolving feelings is enormous. The high value we place on feelings in decision-making is probably the single most important factor to our generation. Indeed, it is difficult for us to make the distinction between calculated thought and instinctive emotion. So self-absorbed are we as passive recipients of emotional appeal through television and movies that it is difficult to imagine going against our feelings in matters where moral integrity seems to dictate direction in our lives.

If previous distant generations tried to be objective, recent generations have rejected objectivity along with the absolutes that define right and wrong. For most people, feelings are the means by which we resolve the crises we face daily. This emotional quicksand was immortalized in the movie series "Star Wars" where the hero, Luke Skywalker, facing crisis after crisis hears the whisper of an inner voice calling him to, "Trust the Force, Luke, go with your feelings." We too hear the force of our own desire whispering to us, "If it feels right, it must be right."

The loss of an objective moral standard in the second half of the twentieth century has made the appeal to emotional satisfaction inevitable. Objective, external standards imposed on personal decision-making are now believed to be oppressive and coercive. The family in our example will feel justified in its decision-making not only on the basis of what is practical, but also on the basis of what feels right to them as a family. Unless they are influenced by an outside objective moral voice of right and wrong, they will make their decision accordingly. It may be a decision to put mother on "life support" or it may be to "allow her to die." In any case it will be practicality and emotional needs rather than reasoned wisdom or mature Christian faith that influence the decision. It is important to realize that even Christians whose faith is genuine and personally important to them may find themselves making decisions more on the basis of practicality and emotional satisfaction than on moral absolutes of right and wrong. We Christians breathe the same air that pollutes the thinking of our contemporaries, and we fail to breathe in deeply the breath of God that cleanses us from the outside and from within.

As Christians we must learn to stand apart from society's approach to ethics and ask ourselves whether there isn't a better word from God in the dilemmas we face in life. Even with a strong Christian faith we will not always make the right decisions, but we live under the grace of God, the promise of the forgiveness of sins, and the presence of the Holy Spirit who works in His holy people to bring about holy lives.

THE PUBLIC ETHIC

Let us consider another interpretation of ethics today. This example is not that of a personal, family crisis, but the crisis of a whole society in which human life itself is at stake for generations to come. In 1993 Congress eliminated procedural obstacles for funding human embryo research and for overthrowing the ban placed on such research by President Reagan in the 1980s. Proposals had been suggested for experimentation to be conducted on *ex utero* (outside the body) embryos. The embryos available, it was said, were leftover ones that had little opportunity for implantation and development into live births because their parents no longer had need of them. Fully human and viable, these embryos were to be used as "lab rats" for the interests of scientists in universities across America. The processes of human embryo research involved manipulation and dissection of human embryos, which when scientists were finished with them, would be discarded as waste material.

When Congress gave approval for resuming research, it supported the National Institute of Health's (NIH) interpretation that these embryos do not have the same moral status as infants and children, saying that they lack sentience and most other qualities considered relevant to the moral status of persons. No particularly convincing argument was made to justify this definition of what an embryo morally is or is not, but no one seemed to notice. NIH simply became its own resource in support of itself. Needless to say, this interpretation by the NIH was akin to having a fox define a code of ethics for the protection of a hen house.

What is of concern here is the way in which ethics and morality are defined in our increasingly utilitarian society. As biased ethicists discussed questions about the ethics of embryo research, they again set the stage for the desired outcome. The way in which the questions were posed set parameters for the debate, eliminating other questions by default. One ethicist raised the question, "Are human embryos so special that not even lifesaving medical benefits can offset the moral cost?" The traditional answer might have been, "Yes, they are!" But in the climate of ethical discussion today, the question was intended to be rhetorical. This same fox of an ethicist then went on to identify the benefits of embryo research in the hen house of science. No existential or spiritual questions were raised or taken seriously by any ethicist within the purview of NIH. Hardly any ethicists apart from the religious community seemed to point out that some things are so horrendous that even public consideration of them offends human dignity.

C. S. Lewis, in many of his science fiction writings, identified the dangers of science when it offers justifications for its projects such as "for the betterment of mankind." It is interesting to realize that personal ethical decision-making seldom considers the long-term effects of a decision, such as the betterment of mankind, because such wisdom dampens the immediate desire for self-gratification. And yet, when public ethical decisions are announced, the appeal to long-term benefit is made to the masses. Perhaps this double standard for ethics works well for us as a nation of people who want freedom to do whatever we want, which is personally gratifying and publicly enhancing.

The personal and public appeal in ethics at this turning of the millennium is nearly always utilitarian in nature. Because of this it is difficult to raise so-called abstract ethical ideas about truth or about the absolutes of right and wrong. The church collectively must come to realize that this is so. It is not enough to complain about ethics today, nor is it appropriate or adequate to politically coerce a nation into passing laws that result in giving an impression that ethics is about that which is legal. Rather, Christians need to bear witness, in their own ethical decision-making, to their faith even when ridiculed for doing so, that others will have a model of the alternative to utilitarianism and emotivism.

Christians must also continue to appeal to reason in the service of faith. Reason offsets emotion, and faith offsets purely utilitarian ethics. Where it is not possible to persuade reasonably, Christians might simply state the truth, take whatever criticism they get for it, and continue to speak the truth in love as the Word of God urges. Christians are not called to success in convincing the world to think differently. We are only called to be faithful, speaking with sensitivity and caring for those whose lives are an empty shell of practical and emotive concerns.

NOTES

[1] I use the words "medical ethics" and "bioethics" as synonyms. Medical ethics is older than bioethics, but Law and Gospel apply to both.

[2] For a book that deals with the practice of spiritual care, readers might well refer to my previous book entitled *Pastoral Care under the Cross: God in the Midst of Suffering* (St. Louis: Concordia Publishing House, 1995).

2

How We Got
to Where We Are

Having briefly described the way in which many people, including Christians, approach ethics today, it is important to point out that ethics has not always been approached in this way. In this chapter we will examine how we came to be the way we are in our decision-making by tracing the development of ethics in history. The foundation on which people have built an ethic has shifted over the centuries, but each shift can be seen in part to be a reaction to the ethics that preceded it. Some of the reaction to previous ways of doing ethics can be seen as a maturity of understanding and a return to truth. Other reactions to previous ethical perspectives might be seen as a societal adolescent rebellion against authority that needs maturing. We may well be living in such an adolescent era today.

To begin, we will look briefly at the philosophical rather than theological development of ethics, saving the latter for the remainder of the book. We will learn from our distant elders how they faced ethical issues in the past. It should be said from the outset that although today's issues present themselves in new technological format, the moral questions are old. The moral issues we face about life and death decision-making are about how we treat human beings in general. These issues have been with us since the beginning, following the Fall into sin and since Cain killed Abel.

We will begin our overview of ethics with what might be called the *classical* or golden age of ethics, stemming from ancient Greece five centuries before Christ. We will examine the classical ethical perspectives of Plato and Aristotle. Whether their influence is accepted or rejected, the ideas of both continue to make an impact on ethics today. From there we will move to what historians now refer to as the *modern* period, the so-called period of Enlightenment of the seventeenth and eighteenth centuries. Immanuel Kant and David Hume will represent this period for our purposes because their influence is still with us today, and yet, their reliance on reason and science is suspect in these *postmodern* times.

The postmodern approach to ethics will be represented by two nineteenth-century philosophers, Søren Kierkegaard and Friedrich Nietzsche. Although these men are not contemporary in our life span they are contemporary in their influence today. Interestingly, Kierkegaard was a Christian and Nietzsche an atheist, but both reacted against the ethics of the modern period. Their influence today is pervasive in the relativism and reaction against absolutes that characterize ethical debate in recent decades.

The presentation of each of these philosophers will be introduced by a contemporary story that illustrates their continuing influence among us today. The reader should be aware that philosophers who follow the *classical* or *modern* thought are not great in number today. The vast majority of people are postmodern in their approach to ethics in choosing to resolve their ethical dilemma according to *what works for them and feels good to them.*

CLASSICAL ETHICS

Terry and Paul had been married for five years. Terry had been on birth control pills for that length of time. Paul had a realistic fear that his family's history of Huntington Disease would be passed on to his offspring and so he was not eager to have children. After someone gave Terry and Paul an article on the availability of donors of sperm, they arranged to see a fertility specialist who suggested that artificial insemination with the use of donor sperm would resolve their genetic problem. But as they drove home, Terry began to have reservations about the idea. She told Paul that it just didn't seem right to her to have another man's sperm father their child. When pressed by Paul, she could not give any explanation for her convictions. She said that it just didn't seem right. Terry went on to say that she had always understood the ideal of marriage and conception to be that a child was meant to be conceived between husband and wife alone. She could not go against this ideal. They eventually adopted a child.

ETHICS BY PLATO

Terry would be called foolishly idealistic by many today for her refusal to make use of donor sperm in order to conceive a child, but she unknowingly represents a classical approach to ethics represented by Plato some twenty-four hundred years ago. Plato believed that the world in which we live is a mere copy of the ideal world and an inferior copy at that. Placing the world of ideals in the spiritual realm, Plato taught that the longing we feel for what is right, good, and true arises from the soul which is a part of that ideal world.[1] Terry was a Platonist in her inexplicable conviction that the ideal was good and anything less than that inferior to it.

The strength of Plato's ethic is that it locates the good in an objective absolute, an ideal. Plato attempted to answer the question, "Where shall we find the good?" There were those, even in Plato's day, who said that it is to be found in one's subjective feelings. Plato responded to the question with the idea of a transcendent world of ideals that gives rise to our reasoned conclusion that there is more to what is good and true than merely our feelings. Subsequent interpretation of Plato's ethics as idealism is ridiculed and rejected by postmodern people. Today idealism is believed to be unrealistic, even a liability in decision-making. How ironic it is that Plato's belief in the *ideal world alone as real* and the physical world as merely its imperfect copy should be reversed in our time by belief in the *physical world alone as real* and the ideal as merely its imperfect reflection.

Plato's world of ideals is a world of absolutes. Ideals as absolutes claim objective reality apart from anything we have to say about them. Contemporary ethics allows little room for discussions of absolutes. Governed for the most part by practicality and emotions, we like to decide on the basis of our feelings what is right and wrong. Plato persuaded the people of his own day to think otherwise, but he does not seem to be convincing many today.

Interestingly, however, individuals often betray their own thirst for objectivity. Although in this age few admit to the existence of absolutes, people nevertheless rely on absolutes when it serves self-interest or, if we are to be more generous in our assessment of human nature, when it reveals a deeper intuitive wisdom. For example, when I tell my students that since they claim there are no absolutes and try to persuade me that moral values are relative, I will therefore randomly assign a failing grade to certain members of the class apart from their performance. They most often rise up immediately in indignation claiming, "That's not fair!" And they are right. What they do not realize is that they are appealing to an objective standard or absolute about what is fair and just. When under pressure, they fall back on the ideal or absolute. Plato would be pleased. Not many self-confessing Platonists reside on ethics committees today, however, and so we can only ferret them out under siege and reveal to them that they share a place on life's stage with Plato after all.

ETHICS BY ARISTOTLE

Kevin's business had taken a bad turn and he was considering filing for bankruptcy. On top of this he had been visiting his eighty-year-old father in the hospital who, for a month, had been disoriented and unable to be fed except through a feeding tube. Supporting a wife and three children on a declining income, Kevin was nevertheless about to send his first child to college in hopes that he could afford to keep him there. Then he was told by the hospital that his father would have to be moved to a nursing home. His father had sufficient funds to pay for care for some years to come, but this would mean the end of Kevin's hope for a financial rescue from his own problems and the end of an inheritance altogether. There was, however, an out. The doctor hinted that the removal of his fathers feeding tube while still in the hospital would put an end to his father's suffering. It would also put an end to Kevin's worries. It was Kevin's call.

No one would blame Kevin for wanting to salvage his business, his son's education, and his own retirement inheritance. To many people with whom Kevin spoke, it seemed pointless to keep up the tube feeding. But Kevin was the one who had to live with the decision he alone was being asked to make. Kevin was a virtuous man. He was honest and wanted to do the right thing regardless of consequences. Perhaps more than anything it mattered to him to act with integrity, so in spite of the threat of financial ruin and all it meant, Kevin refused to withdraw the feeding tube just to secure his own or anyone else's future. Even though his father might linger for weeks, months, or even years, it was Kevin's conviction that his own integrity mattered most. He would face hardship and find satisfaction in knowing he had done the virtuous thing rather than give in to utilitarian concerns. There might be few like Kevin who would have sacrificed practical solutions for personal integrity.

Kevin's claim to integrity as the higher ground is representative of Aristotle's ethics. Aristotle began with the question, "What is it that all people look for in life?" He concluded that the answer was *happiness*. But people seek happiness in the wrong places, he said. It is not found in accumulating wealth or in having good health or even in being able to live without suffering in one's life. Aristotle suggested that real happiness is found in living a life of virtue which aims at the development of moral character. Although character may be difficult for many to define today, Kevin embodied it. In this, Kevin was Aristotelian for valuing his own integrity above his financial security or personal comfort. He could only do so as one who had learned to resist being seduced by the economic temptations to happiness that our society values so highly.

Aristotle's influence continued to draw parameters around the study of ethics until the eighteenth century. Earlier, in the thirteenth century, Thomas Aquinas had so effectively synthesized Christian theology and Aristotelian thought that the ethics of Aristotle dominated both ecclesiastical and civil ethics until the dawn of the Enlightenment. Aristotle's influence on ethics through the formula of what has come to be popularly identified as *The Golden Mean* has served to guide ethical decision-making for generations. It states that the ethical life is one lived virtuously. The virtues are found in seeking the mean—midpoint—between the extremes of excess and deficiency. Courage under pressure, for example, is the *mean* between the excess of foolish impulsiveness and the deficiency of cowardly avoidance.

Aristotle's ethic still appeals to those who believe there is more to life than just getting things done. Many still believe that virtues such as courage, patience, honesty, and reasonable thinking are better ways to deal with difficult medical conditions than the quick fix of emotional reaction. A few ethicists today have proposed, so far unsuccessfully, a return to Aristotle's notion of character development as part of the training of medical professionals who, it is feared, without virtue will tend to pose medical dilemmas and propose solutions in utilitarian or Machiavellian terms.

The intriguing thing about Aristotle's ethic of virtue and character development is that it does not avoid difficult dilemmas. In fact, it requires them, for it is impossible to practice virtue except under circumstances that demand it. Aristotle's ethic is made for those who suffer. In today's world, where suffering is thought to be the worst thing that could happen in illness, it remains to be seen whether anyone will see suffering as an opportunity to practice virtue as the means to develop moral character.

In summary, the classical period of ethics began with the ancient Greeks, the most notable of which were Plato and Aristotle, and served as the foundation for ethics in Western civilization until the Enlightenment of the eighteenth century. Three characteristics are worth remembering. First, classical ethics is characterized by a belief in moral absolutes. The good, the true, and the beautiful are not subjective evaluations made by individuals but possess an ideal and universal reality of their own. Although there have been disagreements among philosophers over the nature of the good, the true, and beautiful, no modern notion of ethics being a matter of individual subjective preference existed. In the past, philosophers were considered explorers intent on discovering the true nature of objective reality.

Second, classical ethics is also characterized by emphasis on character development. In this approach to ethics it is assumed that a good person performs good actions and that good actions produce a good person. Classical ethics, contrary to popular contemporary ethics, rejects the idea that a person can separate what he does from the kind of person he is. One cannot say he is a moral person while living an immoral life. The contemporary attitude may be illustrated by a conversation I overheard between a young woman and her friend in which the young woman said, "Just because I think old people should be refused expensive treatment if they can't pay for it themselves, doesn't mean I am an *uncaring person.*" Separation of the person from his or her attitudes and actions was unthinkable to the Greeks and to classical ethics.

Third, there is no wall between theology and philosophy in the classical ethics of the ancient Greeks. "Mythological and intuitive elements permeate their thinking even where we see the first historical efforts toward conceptualization; they traffic with the old gods even while in the process of coining a new significance for them; and everywhere in the fragments of these … Greeks is the sign of a revelation greater than themselves which they are unveiling for the rest of mankind."[2]

The door was left open by classical ethics for Christian theologians such as Augustine and Aquinas to address ethics in a way that today might be identified as holistic. Classical ethics held center stage until the time of the Enlightenment and what might be called the modern approach to ethics.

MODERN ETHICS

The leap from classical to modern ethics is a leap of about two thousand years—and even that does not bring us to what we usually think of as *modern*, namely our own times. It merely brings us from the influence of the ancient Greeks to the brink of the eighteenth century. Until that time, the Aristotelian approach to ethics virtually dominated western philosophical inquiry. By the end of the sixteenth and beginning of the seventeenth centuries the world had changed sufficiently that philosophers began to question the very foundations of classical thought. We will make our attempt to understand the modern approach to ethics of the eighteenth and nineteenth century in the same way as we did classical ethics. Two stories will be presented, followed by comments on the ethics of Immanuel Kant and David Hume as thinkers of the modern approach to ethics.

Ethics by Kant

Jason, as executive vice president of a large corporation, had come a long way since his boyhood days in Nebraska. Forty-eight years old, single, devoted to his work, and distantly respectful of the religious beliefs of his childhood, Jason now lived in New York City. Severed from the community in which he grew up, he enjoyed the solitude of anonymity in the crowd of business associates that made his life exciting and rewarding.

Following a routine medical examination, it was discovered that Jason had leukemia. Being a rational person, Jason immediately began to make responsible provision for the future and to tie up loose ends involving obligations owed his associates. He had always been admired by these associates for his self-reliance and courage in facing up to things. His physician had said there was a good chance of extending his life a few years through treatment, but both the illness and the treatment would seriously limit his independence and energy level for work. He faced the options of seeking treatment only to delay the inevitable or of rejecting treatment and continuing his present level of activities, which made his life meaningful.

Without consulting friends or associates, he surveyed the dilemma and, in spite of being tempted by his emotions to give in to that which gave his life meaning, decided in favor of treatment, telling himself it was what any reasonable person should do under the circumstances. Jason did not seem to be faced with much of an ethical dilemma. Like many, he decided for himself what he believed to be the best thing to do and did it. He was a self-sufficient, autonomous person who was rational and responsible. He was, even without religion, a moral person. Not many people today are as rational in their ethical decision-making as Jason was in this story.

Jason is the contemporary image of Immanuel Kant. Raised by Christian parents who provided a strong Christian morality, Kant nevertheless rejected the faith of his parents while at the same time retaining Christian morality on the

grounds that such a moral system could be rationally defend-
ed on the basis of natural law. What distinguishes modern
ethics from classical ethics is that modern ethics rejects the
supernatural foundation for ethics while still retaining a concern for moral integrity. Even today we might consider some as
moral persons who categorically reject religion on the grounds
of its irrationality. They tacitly accept the Christian moral system, as did Kant, but unlike Kant they select principles from it
that have a distinctively utilitarian flavor.

The modernism of the eighteenth century passed on to us
the importance of valuing the autonomous individual,
detached from both community and the Christian faith, who
seeks to define ethical behavior on his or her own. We have
inherited from Kant the idea of this autonomous individual
whose authority is his own self-legislating will. For Kant, however, the self-legislating will dare not surrender to the whim of
emotion or utilitarianism as we do today. Because our emotions exercise so strong an influence on us, Kant said, the
demands of reason seem burdensome; therefore we must consider them an obligation or a duty, or we would never follow
them. This sense of duty he referred to as a *sense of oughtness.*
Kant proposed a formula for ethical decision-making: we are
required to act always as if the principle of our individual
action could be universalized as a rule for all people to follow.
In this Kant, was appealing to what has been called *natural law.*

Ethics by Hume

Whitney is Lisa's best friend since childhood. Lisa is married and wants to have children, but is unable to carry them to
full term. She has already experienced three miscarriages in five
years. After discussing the matter with her husband, Lisa
approaches Whitney, who is single, to ask if she will act as surrogate mother for Lisa's child. Whitney is honored and eagerly
agrees to do so, excited about such an experience.
Arrangements are made with an infertility specialist to pro-

ceed, when Whitney's mother questions the wisdom of her acting as surrogate mother. When asked by her mother for her reasons for agreeing to the arrangement, Whitney says, "Lisa is my friend and I like her. She has suffered enough with miscarriages and this is my way to bring her some happiness into her life."

Whitney and Lisa also agree that it feels like the right thing to do for all concerned. Both women admit to personal feelings as the most important indicator of what is right and wrong. Unlike Jason the Kantian who valued rational, universal principles of morality, here emotion is highly prized and actually serves as the foundation of moral choice for Whitney and Lisa. They are convinced that what they feel deeply justifies their behavior, regardless of objections or obstacles that might arise.

Like Whitney and Lisa, many people today owe their justification for reliance on feelings in ethical decision-making to David Hume. Hume said that morality is more properly felt than judged. Widely known for his attacks on Christianity, Hume reasoned that there is no way to prove the existence of the supernatural. But he was skeptical about reliance on rational thought as well. All that could be trusted were "feelings, not knowing." As one who excluded spiritual belief from ethics, Hume might well be called the father of *feel-good ethics*. At the root, he said, all men value moral ideas merely for their agreeableness; ethics is nothing more than the likes and dislikes of people, and such likes and dislikes are merely the result of the avoidance of pain and the pursuit of pleasure. The value we assign to emotional satisfaction in decision-making today is enormous. The contemporary tendency to justify morality on the basis of feelings found a footing in the birth and rise of psychology in the latter part of the nineteenth century.

More needs to be said about the place of feelings in ethics, but now it is time to turn to the thought of Søren Kierkegaard and Friedrich Nietzsche to see how reactions to Hume's ideas were carried to further conclusions, resulting in postmodernism's ultimate inability to determine moral value in anything apart from emotional satisfaction.

In summary, the approach to the modern period of ethics is characterized first by the rejection of external authority, particularly the spiritual authority of Christianity. The biblical foundation of ethics that had guided the world for seventeen centuries was lost. The loss was experienced first among philosophers and later sifted down to the wider population. Without divine origins, ethics began to be defined by rationalism, utilitarianism, and emotivism. Ethics, separated from biblical morality, gave way to what works and what feels good as determined by the individual.

The second characteristic of the modern approach to ethics is that it centered in the autonomy of the individual. The ideal man was believed to be the individual who viewed life rationally, not spiritually. Hume, who gave ethics over to the emotive and was skeptical of reason, was even more skeptical of belief in the spiritual realities. The rise of science during the eighteenth and nineteenth centuries provided the model for a reconstruction of ethics. Following the paradigm of scientific proofs, ethics began to be defined by pragmatic experimentation with outcomes. That is, ethics began to be defined by the success or failure of results.

Kant, not being a utilitarian, proposed as the basis for ethics the existence of universal moral principles accessible by reason, not faith. Reason as the only source of ethics became to philosophy what the laws of nature had become to science. Ethics gradually separated from the transcendent absolutes of classical ethics and, unaided by such absolutes or faith, became reliant on the new absolute—reason.

POSTMODERN ETHICS

It is strange to speak of something as being postmodern when the word modern is seemingly descriptive of the most current state of affairs. Postmodern sounds like a contradiction in terms, but it is descriptive of ideas that succeeded the modern. We have already defined the modern as emerging at a particular time in history and lasting for nearly three hundred years. Postmodern times may be said to have begun in this country about the middle of the twentieth century, following World War II. We live in postmodern times today which, of course, are experienced by us as contemporary. The postmodern approach to ethics is a reaction to the modern approach just as the modern was a reaction to the classical approach before it. It is both very complicated and very simple at the same time. The two philosophers most influential in the birth of postmodern thought are Søren Kierkegaard and Friedrich Nietzsche. To proceed, we begin again with two stories and follow with commentaries on Kierkegaard and Nietzsche.

Ethics by Kierkegaard

Andrea and Scott became engaged after dating for a year and a half. They lived in a Midwestern town of less than six hundred people and were actively involved in their church, one attended by almost everyone in town. The congregation was a good place for business connections in the community, but no other opportunity for social life was available. Being raised in a community that regarded sex before marriage as a sin, Scott and Andrea had nevertheless become intimate. Ultimately, Andrea became pregnant. Immediate marriage seemed an easy way to hide the unexpected pregnancy, but Andrea resisted Scott's suggestion of an earlier wedding date. Andrea wanted to determine her own future and did not want to feel pressured into early marriage merely as a way to avoid the community's discovery of her pregnancy. She wanted to make her own choice in the matter apart from outside pressures.

Andrea confided to Scott that she was considering abortion. She was disappointed when Scott quickly supported the idea and suggested that it would be better than having to face the judgment of the church and community. Feeling more alone than ever, Andrea decided to go away by herself for a few days to think things through and make a decision for herself.

When she returned she told Scott that she had decided to have the baby and that she wanted a small, quiet wedding on the original date they had chosen, three months away. Scott initially resisted but finally supported her decision.

Such a commonplace situation hardly seems to call for a moral crisis in a contemporary environment where abortion is legal and generally socially acceptable. Scott's acceptance of Andrea's *right* to make her own decision, even though he was the father of her child, is supported by civil law. Andrea represents a postmodern interpretation of Kierkegaard's emphasis on the importance of each person taking responsibility for his or her own decisions and being free of external coercion in order to do so. The ethical life, Kierkegaard said, is the decisive life in which one faces up to the decision of the moment. To avoid making a decision is to have a decision made for us.

Kierkegaard lived in Denmark during the second half of the nineteenth century in a small community that centered its life outwardly on the church. Because of what Kierkegaard observed as the apathy and lack of authenticity of the many who went to church regularly, he "set himself the task of determining whether Christianity can still be lived or whether a civilization still nominally Christian must finally confess spiritual bankruptcy." His wrestling with this question took on personal dimensions as he discovered not only authentic faith, but also concluded that in relationship to God we are always in the wrong. He came to see every ethical decision as a crisis of faith and concluded that indecisiveness in moral decision-making is in reality an unwillingness to face up to God. To not face up to God is to be apathetic and unethical. Being decisive, he said, brings us face-to-face with God where authenticity puts us on our knees before Him. Decisiveness and the importance of choice as a matter of faith were sovereign for Kierkegaard.

Andrea's decisiveness unfolded in the context of her personal faith in God and showed itself in her decision not to have the abortion and not to hide the sin, which led to her pregnancy. According to Kierkegaard, Andrea is an authentic and therefore ethical person. Today the emphasis on choice as the central doctrine of contemporary ethics is perched precariously in the void that once was filled by Kierkegaard's Christian faith.

ETHICS BY NIETZSCHE

Anthony had been battling metastatic bone cancer for about a year when he called his doctor and asked for a prescription pain reliever that clearly exceeded the therapeutic dosage he had had in the past. Indirectly he conveyed to his doctor that he had every intention of taking the medication to end his life. With some hesitancy his doctor agreed to authorize the prescription, believing it was Anthony's decision, not his own, that was paramount. Anthony was a fifty-three-year-old divorced businessman with no living children. Feeling alone one night, he had confided in his friend John about his plans. John immediately conveyed his disapproval, giving as his reasons that all life belongs to God and that it is not our prerogative to end a life at will.

Anthony stiffened at John's reply and attacked what he believed was the motive for his disapproval. He said John was imposing his own values on Anthony's life and was doing so for selfish reasons. As far as Anthony was concerned, it was a powerplay on John's part to prevent Anthony from prematurely depriving John of the benefits derived from Anthony as his business associate. Hurt by Anthony's interpretation of his motives, John retreated from further comment on the matter and tried to repair the damage to their friendship by half-heartedly supporting Anthony's right to make up his own mind. Anthony represents Nietzsche's thought that ethics is merely a game of power in which the stronger attempts to dominate the weaker.

Not many in these postmodern times assume any longer that there is objective moral truth such as that proclaimed by the Christian view of reality. All ethics is merely a matter of one person trying to impose his own opinions on another. Ethics, in short, is a mask for power. On this assumption, different viewpoints about moral issues are acceptable so long as no one point of view claims to be universally true for all. Privately a person may believe what he or she wishes, but publicly it is no longer acceptable to attempt to persuade others that one view is right and another is wrong. The debate over abortion in this country has been stalled for decades because the pro-choice side accuses the pro-life side of merely using ethics as a political power play. Years of impasse instead of compromise on what even many pro-choice people agree is an atrocity, namely partial birth abortion, is illustrative of this. Any compromise is seen as a weakness in the struggle for power.

Since Nietzsche did not believe in God and saw Christianity as an interference with a person's natural inclination to aggression, he concluded that morality was simply Christianity's way of controlling the behavior of others according to its own standard. Observing what he believed to be the waning power of Christianity in the world, he concluded that the hypocrisy he observed among Christians meant that even they no longer believed in God. Nietzsche therefore announced the *death of God*. He suggested that any man with courage enough would admit the same. Continuing his attack, Nietzsche said Christianity was a sickness in need of a cure, something which could be accomplished by eliminating its influence in Western civilization. From Nietzschian thought comes the deconstruction of all western ideas that have been heavily shaped by Christianity, ethics included. Since for Nietzsche all ethics is about power, in place of traditional morality he proposed an ethic where the *superman* (the man above the distinction between good and evil) unashamedly exercises his own *will to power* over the weaker man (still inhibited by morality distinctions). This alone would free people to live beyond the designations of good and evil proposed by Christianity.

In summary, the approach to the postmodern period of ethics is characterized by three factors. First, it rejects the rational search for an ethic characteristic of the modern approach. This is one of the reasons it is impossible to have a reasoned debate on the floor of Congress or in the classroom over abortion since rationality itself has come under attack. Just as modern ethics rejected the spiritual in favor of the rational, so postmodern ethics rejects the rational, believing that what is claimed as truth is merely personal opinion or an excuse for the exercise of power. In rejecting the rational, postmodern people are left with little more than a visceral response to ethical issues.

The second characteristic of postmodern ethics centers on the autonomous individual and his expectation of tolerance on the part of the community for the choices he makes. Postmodern people no longer find it acceptable to make moral judgments on the behavior of others. Freedom from *restraint* and for the *right to choose* is of the highest importance. This interpretation of freedom is one way of dealing with pluralism in our society. It is usually accompanied by the dismantling of Christian influence in ethics. Even those with a sincere personal Christian faith may be seduced into accepting the postmodern interpretation of ethics which allows no limits that inhibit the rights of the individual in defining moral choices.

Third, postmodern ethics is characterized by the *loss of objective meaning* to ethics. Since postmodernism allows for no transcendent, objective meaning in life, it follows that ethics can have no objective moral meaning either; therefore, all ethics is subjective and meaningless except in so far as each person creates his or her own meaning. What is right for one may not be right for another, depending on what it means to each person. No debate can take place over ethical issues because, without objective meanings, whatever is said is simply opinion which carries no authority except for the individual expressing it. However, the postmodern approach to ethics, which has left our society with nothing more than relativity and subjectivity, is beginning to show signs of disintegration. There appears to be a hunger for more objective meaning and truth in the younger generation. A foundational story, we will see, is where meaning can be found.

Notes

[1] Plato's ideals might be understood to correspond to what we mean by absolutes.

[2] William Barrett, *The Irrational Man* (New York: Anchor Books/Doubleday, 1958), p. 5.

3

A Foundational Story
for Ethics

In the classical approach, ethics began with a foundation that integrated both human reason and transcendent realities. In the modern approach to ethics, the transcendent was discarded. The postmodern approach abandoned reason. Having lost both the transcendent and the reasonable, there is no objective meaning or objective content to ethics today, leaving each person to create his or her own subjective meaning and morality. Unless we are to be reduced to a society in which there are no moral limits other than that which each individual chooses to create for himself, we must again seek a reasonable and transcendent meaning that will guide us in how we are to live together.

THE STORY

As we have already seen, ethics can be built on the ideal, the virtuous, the dutiful, the utilitarian, and the emotive. But there is a more basic and more enduring foundation on which to establish ethics. Ethics needs a story to give it purpose and meaning. The realization that *story* is crucial as a basis for ethics has re-emerged in the search for a way out of the moral chaos. Story gives coherent meaning to our life together. Christians recognize the Story—the Bible—as the original foundation of our common life as human beings under God.

A common story has a beginning, a middle, and an end. This narrative structure ties together all the parts into a meaningful whole. All stories attempt to make sense of the raw material of knowledge and experience that would otherwise be perceived merely as random data. Stories are powerful because they give coherence to our lives and affect the way we think and act. The transforming power of a story can be illustrated in the example of marriage.

As an only child, I spent a great deal of time alone. I do not recall feeling lonely, however, and my introspective hours seemed to increase my capacity for imagination and creativity. I had many neighborhood friends who became my surrogate siblings as I needed them. At age sixteen I came to the conviction that I was called to enter the ministry. After eight years of college and seminary, I graduated and was ordained. When called to serve as pastor of my first congregation, I was not married.

Two years later I met and married Susan. Each of us made the adaptations and changes required of living with a spouse, as well as the transition from living for self to living for someone else. For the first time in my life I began to make the sacrifices demanded of a loving marriage relationship. My priorities for ministry changed as a result of being a husband and, later, a father. After John and Mary were born, as necessity demanded, our lives focused more on their needs than on ours. At the end of a particularly exhausting day, when the children still needed help with homework or wanted me to attend some activity at school, I remember wondering if I would ever again experience the solitude of my bachelor years.

But as the years passed I realized that the solitude I now craved was not one I desired to spend alone. The solitude I had come to enjoy and need was the solitude of time spent with my wife. She and I often took long walks during which we thought through the challenges of the day, sorted out our misunderstandings, worked out our future plans, and prayed silently together as we walked.

I could never return to the experience of solitude from earlier in life, nor do I wish to do so. The relationship of marriage itself has transformed my desires and needs. I can no longer think or behave in a way that excludes my marriage as a consideration of all that I am and do. The story of our marriage has shaped my wife and me and continues to deepen the mystery of our life together.

My wife and I have intentionally agreed to some *rules* about how we communicate our disagreements, how we might best be supportive of one another, and what we need to do to keep our spiritual life in focus. But it is not the rules themselves that have changed us. The rules set the parameters within which the *relationship* developed and shaped us. Marriage as the story of a relationship which shapes us mirrors our collective relationship with God and illustrates the difference between ethical behavior lived under Law (rules) and ethical behavior lived as a result of the life-changing power of the Gospel.

A story, such as that which unfolds in marriage, changes lives and pulls together the loose ends, giving coherent meaning to life. Another kind of story is told by elderly people who are terminally ill; it is one in which they often rehearse the past experiences of their lives. They seek to pull together the pieces in order to discover the truth about themselves so they can die in peace. As human beings we seem to know inherently that there is more to life than the chaos that surrounds us.

In these postmodern times, however, it is difficult for us to understand and experience a story that is larger than our personal stories. We value autonomy as the highest good and find little encouragement in the culture to look outside ourselves for meaning and direction. Yet we need the larger Story of which our personal stories are a part. Our need to be part of that larger Story is so strong that we are sometimes drawn into fictitious stories, mere *virtual reality,* that seem at the moment to offer what we are looking for. As such, we are drawn into soap operas, unfolding stories in the nightly news, and portrayals of lives produced on stage, imagining what it would be like to be part of something more than our bleak and lonely lives—part of a larger story that resolves the confusion and uncovers the real truth. We get caught up superficially in these virtual reality portrayals that seem to touch an emptiness in us. We sense that we are out of touch with the real Story that is larger than our own personal story.

Our individual stories lack the framework of a larger Story into which all our lives fit together meaningfully. The Bible tells the real, larger Story that we seek. The Bible is *The Story* God tells that gives meaning to our lives together with him and with one another. I am aware that the word "story" in our time is almost always associated with fiction, but God's Story is the ultimate, true Story. The Story God tells is a historical narrative, a true story still in the telling. Christians speak of the Bible as the inspired and infallible Word of God. It is in this sense that I speak of the Bible as Story.

THE STORY GOD TELLS

The Story God tells is full of mystery. It is not a story that provides an answer to every question that we might ask. The truth is that we often ask the wrong questions. God's Story is a story that provides only what we need to learn to fear, love, and trust in God and to live together faithfully. The Bible speaks of Jesus as the focal point of God's mystery story.

> Great indeed, we confess, is the mystery of our religion:
> He was manifested in the flesh, vindicated in the Spirit,
> seen by angels, preached among the nations, believed
> on in the world, taken up in glory. (1 Timothy 3:16)

The Sherlock Holmes stories are not really mysteries, for they turn out at the end of the book to have an explanation that resolves any mystery that might have confronted us at the beginning. Someone has said that the difference between the words "mystery" and "secret" is that a secret once revealed is no longer a secret but that a mystery revealed only leads deeper into itself and is never fully resolved.[1] When the secret of a "whodunit" is solved by Sherlock Holmes, the secret is told. There is no more secret. But when God tells His Story about the mystery of life, there is no limit to its depth and grandeur. It is unfathomable. It keeps on revealing truth in each generation, so that all lives are drawn into the one Story God tells.

God's mystery Story reveals enough for us to know what we need to know in order to live meaningfully in this life and with certainty toward the life to come. The Story is about God first of all. It is about the God revealed as Father, Son, and Holy Spirit. The facts of the Story are easy to tell, but the mystery is revealed only to people of faith. Briefly told, the Story is that God made the world and all that is in it and declared it all to be *good*. But something, not of God's doing, went wrong so that the world now can now only be described as a corrupted good. That corruption is deep and cannot be overcome by human beings. In what went wrong, death entered the picture and continues to eat away at us like a slowly advancing cancer needing a cure, a victory over death. That need was fulfilled in Jesus' death on the cross for all people.

The world went wrong when, having been given the freedom by God to love or reject him as our Maker, our first parents challenged God and chose rebellion. Not satisfied with having been created in the *image of God*, Adam and Eve wanted to *be* God. The rebellion in the Garden of Eden tells of the disobedience as centering on the desire to experience not only the good God had given, but also the evil he had not. This desire was not merely one of curiosity but at the core was an act of rebellion. It is the ongoing rebellion and resulting alienation from God that has infected every generation that has ever lived.

That portion of God's Story called the Old Testament reveals God's work in planning and executing the reconciliation necessary to restore our relationship with God. Because God is good He still wants the best for us, the good for us. But human rebellion always resists it. God's continual making of covenants with His people and the people's repeated breaking of their relationship with God runs through the Old Testament. It is the record of human fierceness and hard-heartedness, and of God's unfailing goodness.

The portion of God's Story called the New Testament is the fulfillment of the Old Testament. It speaks of God's plan being carried out in reconciling us through His Son, Jesus Christ. It is by faith in Jesus Christ that human beings are restored and reconciled to God. God's people find their assurance of reconciliation in the forgiveness of sins through Christ, and they live in a new relationship with God. In becoming reconciled to the holy God by faith in Jesus, we become a holy people. How we live is the topic of ethics for Christians. In Christ, holy people live holy lives.

STORY, CREEDS, AND LITURGY

The details of God's Story are found in the Bible, from *Genesis* through *Revelation.* Early in the history of the church the Story was summarized in the Apostles' Creed, the Nicene Creed, and the Athanasian Creed. Creeds are the collective witness the church has made to the world. The earliest of the church's creeds, the Apostles' Creed, confesses faith in Jesus:

> I believe in ... Jesus Christ ... who was conceived by the Holy Spirit, born of the virgin Mary, suffered under Pontius Pilate, was crucified, died and was buried. He descended into hell. The third day he rose again from the dead. He ascended into heaven and sits at the right hand of God the Father Almighty. From thence he will come to judge the living and the dead.

Creeds are the church's way of speaking the mystery of God in succinct form against those who distort God's Story in every generation. The New Testament itself sometimes expresses the Story in creeds: statements of the collective orthodox faith of the church. One of these creeds proclaims the message of Jesus Christ clearly:

> Have this mind among yourselves, which you have in Christ Jesus, who, though he was in the form of God, did not count equality with God a thing to be grasped, but emptied himself, taking the form of a servant, being born in the likeness of men. And being found in human form he humbled himself and became obedient unto death, even death on a cross. Therefore God has highly exalted him and bestowed on him the name which is above every name, that at the name of Jesus every knee should bow, in heaven and on earth and under the earth, and every tongue confess that Jesus Christ is Lord, to the glory of God the Father. (Philippians 2:5–11)

Another place the mystery Story of God is told is in the liturgy of the church's worship, which has roots in biblical times. Preparation for hearing the mystery God reveals begins with Confession and Absolution. Forgiveness opens the door for us to stand before God who is holy. The pastor speaking God's words from the New Testament begins, "If we confess our sins, God, who is faithful and just, will forgive our sins and cleanse us from all unrighteousness."[2]

> Together therefore the worshipers confess their sins:
>
> Most merciful God, we confess that we are by nature sinful and unclean. We have sinned against you in thought, word and deed, by what we have done and by what we have left undone. We have not loved you with our whole heart; we have not loved our neighbors as ourselves. We justly deserve your present and eternal punishment. For the sake of your Son, Jesus Christ, have mercy on us. Forgive us, renew us, and lead us, so that we may delight in your will and walk in your ways to the glory of your holy name. Amen.[3]

The absolution or pronouncement of forgiveness is then given by the pastor who speaks in behalf of God:

Almighty God in his mercy has given his Son to die for
you and for his sake forgives you all your sins. As a
called and ordained servant of the Word I therefore forgive you all your sins in the Name of the Father and of
the Son and of the Holy Spirit....

It is the Word of God that forgives sins and not the pastor, but when God's Word is spoken by the pastor, forgiveness
takes place.

The liturgy continues with the Word of God heard in
both the Bible readings and the sermon. The New Testament
says, "The Word became flesh and dwelt among us." That
incarnate Word is identified as Jesus. God is indeed present
among us in the Word that is heard from the altar. The high
point of the liturgy comes when we are invited to come for-
ward and participate in the meal God has provided for us. It is
a small feast, a taste of the heavenly banquet yet to come. In
the Lord's Supper God feeds us with Jesus' body and blood, all
of which makes sense only as the fulfillment of the Old
Testament sacrificial system. The feeding of God's people is
prefaced with the words:

Our Lord Jesus Christ, on the night when he was
betrayed, took bread, and when he had given thanks,
he broke it and gave it to his disciples and said: Take,
eat; this is my body, which is given for you. This do in
remembrance of me. In the same way also he took the
cup after supper, and when he had given thanks, he
gave it to them, saying: Drink of it, all of you; this is my
blood of the new testament, which is shed for you for
the forgiveness of sins. This do, as often as you drink of
it, in remembrance of me.[4]

The "remembrance" is not merely a recalling of events
long ago, but it is also an ongoing experience that Christ has
given us and continues to give us until the end of time. Jesus'
expression "do this" means that we are to continue to "eat"
and "drink" of it as God continues to come to us in His body
and blood today. Jesus continues to come to His people as He
did in the first supper in the upper room on the night before

He died. He continues to feed us with Himself as the bread of heaven. In this body and blood of the Word made flesh, heaven comes down to earth, and in worship we stand in the presence of God's holiness. It is a hidden Presence: hidden in bread and wine. The mystery of God's work continues in the mystery of the Holy Communion. Worship is not so much our service of praise to God (although we respond with praise to what God does) as it is God's serving us in Word and Sacrament each Sunday (Sunday being the day Jesus rose from the dead). In the worship service, God reconciles us to Himself through the forgiveness of sins so that we might stand in His holy presence as His holy people. As His holy people we have access to Him and are invited by God to bring our petitions to Him. Having been served by God at the altar, we leave to enter the world where our service to God begins. We serve God in many ways, not the least of which is in the decisions we make about matters of life and death.

The world calls this ethics. Christians call it living holy lives as holy people. This is the Story God has been revealing since the beginning of time. In this story we begin to uncover some of the meaning of the ethical life we are called to live as the holy people of God.

NOTES

[1] I am indebted to John Kleinig, Dean of the Chapel and professor at Luther Seminary, North Adelaide, Australia, for this understanding of mystery and secret.

[2] Adapted from 1 John 1:8–9, the liturgy reflects the invitation of God's story to repent.

[3] Divine Service II, *Lutheran Worship* (St. Louis: Concordia Publishing House, 1982) p. 158.

[4] *Lutheran Worship*, p. 171.

4

Holy People, Holy Lives

WHO WE ARE AND WHAT WE DO

The word *ethics* seems to have originated with the ancient Greeks and described not merely a person's behavior, but also his character. Human character is, among other things, what distinguishes us from the animals and calls us to behave in ways that produce such virtues as justice, compassion, courage, and integrity.

Men of both the ancient Greek worldview and the biblical worldview probed the question, "What is man?" The ancient Greek philosophers looked for answers in the natural world around them, while the writers of the Bible found their answer in the revealed Word of God spoken through patriarchs, prophets, and finally in the Word which became flesh and lived among us, Jesus. The psalm writer in the Old Testament was overwhelmed with God's creation of mankind saying, "What is man that you are mindful of him, or the son of man that you care for him? You made him a little lower than the heavenly beings and crowned him with glory and honor." (Psalm 8:4–5 NIV)

How you think about ethics will depend on your answer to the question, "What is man?" If a human being is merely a part of nature and is nothing more than physical, mental, and emotional parts, then a person's behavior or ethic will be guided by the practical, rational, or emotional, respectively. But if a human being is more than the sum of these parts and if men and women are created "a little lower than the angels" and are sustained by, and responsible to, the holy God, then human life and ethics will be guided by deeper spiritual meanings found in relationship with God.

The meaning of words change with time and new contexts. Today the word *ethics* is used less and less as an indicator of a person's character and more and more to describe his actions. In a strange twist of postmodern irrationality, it can now be said that actions have nothing to do with the kind of person one is. This was recently illustrated in an interview with a young woman who had been arrested for attempted murder when she dumped her newborn infant into a garbage can and left the infant outside in sub-zero weather to die. The attorneys and jurors, sympathetic to the young mother, wanted to make it clear to the world that, in spite of their finding her guilty, "this doesn't mean she is a bad person." Can one be a person of good character and kill her newborn infant simply because it is an inconvenient time to raise a child? Or is there something deeply wrong with such murderous human behavior? Our society is one small step away from excusing this kind of irresponsible behavior since we have already crossed the line from viewing ethics as having to do with character to ethics as choices and actions divorced from the person *as* person.

In the latter half of the twentieth century, ethics had more to do with freedom to choose what I wish to choose. Emphasis is on the choosing, not on the one who chooses. What matters is not what is chosen, but the right to choose. The public debate over abortion and euthanasia has been illustrative of this view of ethics. Ethics in these postmodern times has come to be understood as the right to choose, not how to choose the right.

THE QUESTION

What is it that we are trying to define when we speak of ethics? Is it the person or one's actions? Can they be separated? The ancient Greeks and most of the civilized world thought it impossible to separate the behavior of a person from the character of a person. Recall Aristotle, who believed that development of character was the aim of ethics and demonstrated the building of character through virtuous living, thus "we become good by doing good." Aristotle's *doctrine of the mean* was a formula for learning to identify and implement the practice of virtue. On this Aristotelian foundation, the medieval theologian Thomas Aquinas constructed the moral theology of the church for the late Middle Ages. From the Thomistic amalgam of philosophy and theology, *canon law* evolved, distinguishing actions that are moral from those that are not. Aquinas set the church on a course that eventually moved the focus of morality off the person and on to his behavior. As a result both Catholics and Protestants have come to view ethics as following moral prescriptions for right actions. They have responded to the question "What is ethics?" by answering that it is about moral prescriptions for right behavior.

When ethics is reduced to following rules for right behavior, being sure to follow the right rule to the letter becomes paramount. But what if ethics is not entirely about behavior alone or acting according to rules? What if ethics is first of all about the kind of person I am? What if the primary question becomes not, What is a moral *action?* but, What is a moral *person?* The absence of the latter question in our time ought to concern us as Christians. Jesus said, "A tree is recognized by its fruit" (Matthew 12:33), and again, "Blessed are the pure in heart" (Matthew 5:8).

Indeed, the tree is known by its fruit—but not always. We do not challenge the words of Jesus here, but we qualify them the way Jesus did when He also said, "Blessed are the pure in heart." Ethical behavior that is the product of a pure heart is the fruit of the Spirit of God. But even as Christians we are still people who are by nature part of an imperfect and fallen world. Even the pure in heart are not perfect, nor are they omnipotent or omniscient. We don't always know what is right and we don't always do what is right. Further, if in defining morality by our outward actions we believe we have acted morally, then we will see no reason to repent when we have done what we think is right. It is not uncommon for people, even for Christians, to do the right thing for the wrong reasons. It is no secret that we human beings can deceive both ourselves and others by choosing the right while being in the wrong, that is, having the wrong motivations.

Consider the case of Angela: Angela was asked by the doctor to approve the withdrawal of life support from her sister's lifeless body. Her sister was clearly clinically dead. But seeing her sister's lungs rise and fall with every artificial breath of the respirator, Angela was not convinced of it. She asked for time to think about the decision. Some hours later she told the doctor that she wanted the life support systems withdrawn because, she said, "I can't bear to see my sister suffer any longer." Angela made the right choice but for the wrong reason. In truth, her reason had more to do with her own unwillingness to bear what she believed to be her sister's suffering than with what was morally right or wrong about what she believed to be the willful taking of her sister's life.

We might say that Angela did no wrong, because she misunderstood the situation. Her sister was indeed already clinically dead. But Angela did not believe this. As far as Angela was concerned, she was being given the choice between life and death, and that did not trouble her. What troubled her was having to bear the burden of what she believed to be her sister's suffering. The point of Angela's story is that making even the right choice does not necessarily mean we are in the right.

Recall Kierkegaard's words, "In relation to God we are always in the wrong." Indeed we are, until we come under the grace of God. Angela might well have shot her sister with a gun the week before when her sister was still lucid but in pain, rather than see her suffer. Then it might have been more clearly seen that Angela both did the wrong thing and also has a questionable moral character.

A NEW LANGUAGE

Because the word *ethics* has lost all substantive meaning and in itself has begun to contribute to today's moral confusion, it is time for Christians to think, at least for use among themselves, in terms of a new language. This language is new to us, although ancient in origin; it is the language of *holiness* in the Story that God tells.

The foundation of holiness language is God's introduction of Himself to Moses saying: "Say to all the congregation of the people of Israel, You shall be holy; for I the Lord your God am holy" (Leviticus 19:2).

The Bible does not define the holiness of God, but it does spell out the meaning and implications of the holiness of God's people. God's people are called holy in the Old Testament because of their proximity to the holy God. They have access to Him through the name He revealed to them on Mt. Sinai, and they are able to stand before God in the worship and ritual sacrifices inaugurated by God on Sinai, which anticipated the sacrifice of Christ on the cross. The Story God tells describes how He created for Himself a holy people, distinct from all the people of the earth. In an encounter with God, the Lord said to Moses:

> Thus you shall say to the house of Jacob, and tell the people of Israel: You have seen what I did to the Egyptians, and how I bore you on eagles' wings and brought you to myself. Now therefore, if you will obey

my voice and keep my covenant, you shall be my possession among all peoples; for all the earth is mine, and you shall be to me a kingdom of priests and a holy nation. (Exodus 19:3–6)

When we call someone such as Mother Teresa holy, we usually have in mind the *moral* quality of her life: qualities of mercy, compassion, and general goodness. The word *holy* in the Bible describes God, not as to His moral character, but as to His essence or being. "I AM WHO I AM" is the name God gives to Himself. Without God being who He is, even our own *being* would be a mystery to us. An increasing number of people today fail to grasp the meaning of life and consequently have no idea how to live rightly. It is only in relationship to God that a human's *being* becomes meaningful. In the New Testament, Paul points out to Greek philosophers in Athens that one of their own poets came close to the truth when he wrote, "In him [God] we live and move and *have our being*" (Acts 17:28).

Holiness is the language of relationship with God. More of the Story unfolds as Moses asks to see God face-to-face:

Moses said, "I pray thee, show me thy glory." [And God] said, "I will make all my goodness pass before you, and will proclaim before you my name 'The Lord'; and I will be gracious to whom I will be gracious, and will show mercy on whom I will show mercy. But," he said, "you cannot see my face; for man shall not see me and live" (Exodus 33:18–20).

Moses asked to see God's glory, as a sign of His holiness, His *being*. Yet God refused on the grounds that it is not possible for any human being to see the holy God and survive the experience. God offered Moses, instead, His goodness. It is from this revelation of God's goodness that we begin to glimpse the meaning of the word *good*, "I will be gracious, and will show mercy."

In the New Testament Jesus affirms the revelation at Sinai that "only God is good" (Luke 18:19). Since the time of the Greek philosophers, people have tried to define and locate the good. Plato, Aristotle, and others, as close as they may or may not have come, never found it. Good is known only by those who are God's holy people, those to whom God chooses to reveal it.

Although God created human beings as good, in this fallen world good is always a corrupted good. Pure goodness cannot come from the mind or feelings of a human being. It comes from God. We begin to understand ethics and morality rightly once we realize that it is not what we define as good that matters, but what God says is good that counts. Ethics or morality is not something we create, but something God has given us.

God's holy people live under God's goodness. As the measure of morality, goodness is not *derived* from behavior but is *reflected* in the behavior of the redeemed, by grace through faith in Christ. God revealed His holy presence through Moses to the weak and helpless people He had brought out of slavery in Egypt. After God told Moses His plans for making them His holy people, He gave them laws to protect their holiness. If they violated the laws, they defiled themselves and could no longer stand in God's holy presence until they had ritually been made holy again through forgiveness. This happened repeatedly in the Old Testament as sacrifices had to be offered morning and evening for the sins of the people. But God was only halfway through His Story in the Old Testament. The real good was yet to come. When it arrived, it came in flesh and blood with the name of Jesus.

So we have returned to where we started. We began with the question, "Does being moral mean doing moral actions or being a moral person?" As evidence of the difficulty in answering this question, we have called attention to the fact that it is possible to do the right thing for the wrong reason. And we have also made a case for the fact that morality must begin with the transformation of the person, and only then might the possibility of moral actions follow. We have concluded with a new way of speaking of morality through the language of God's holiness and His goodness.

Being and Doing

We need to understand how the *being* of a person can become separated from the *doing* or actions of a person. Our examination of Sin will show how this happens. It will help us understand the origins of the problem we face in bioethics today. Surveying the entire field of morality will help us understand that ethics is not merely about avoiding the muddles but about gaining the ultimate victory over Sin. God's Story reveals the realities of life's muddy field, the puddles, and the ultimate goal. To put it theologically, the Bible reveals the heart of the problem which is Sin and the goal which is ultimate victory over *sin, death, and the devil.*

Who We Are and What We Do

I cannot remember when someone other than my wife or children said to me, "I'm sorry." Outside of those closest to me, what eludes my memory even more is the response, appropriate to an apology, "I forgive you." Neither confession of wrongdoing nor words of forgiveness are heard much anymore. The absence of opportunity for confession and absolution in matters of life and death decision-making in medicine, for example, seems to leave medical ethics outside the realm of moral examination. Living in an increasingly amoral culture we are less and less willing to identify behavior that, until a few years ago, was clearly recognized as crossing the line. Today we are unwilling even to speak of sin and the need for forgiveness in our lives, and yet it is killing us not to do so.

It is not hard to understand why we no longer know where to draw the line in issues of bioethics or any other ethical issues for that matter. We are no longer sure of any clear distinction between good and evil, between right and wrong. Although one may argue with this, I suspect there is more truth in it than we like to admit. Why do we fail to distinguish between good and evil, right and wrong, in issues of bioethics?

I once asked a group of people to tell me the reasons for their hesitancy to make such moral judgments. With a bit of hesitancy they were able to identify two reasons for their reluctance. The first was the discomfort they felt with what they believed to be an arbitrary distinction between judging a person's behavior and judging that person himself. It was hard for them to believe that it is really possible to "love the sinner and hate the sin." These students were therefore content to judge neither the person nor his behavior, being more mistakenly amenable to the biblical injunction, "first take the log out of your own eye, and then you will see clearly to take out the speck that is in your brother's eye" (Luke 6:42). They chose to make a judgment neither about their own log nor their neighbor's speck.

There was more to their hesitancy than the distinction between person and behavior. After all, the distinction between *the kind of person I am and the actions I perform* is something postmodern people make all the time. The group expressed a reluctance to make even the slightest judgment against what they clearly communicated in non-verbal ways as wrong, even repulsive.

A second reason for their hesitancy regarding moral judgments was the fear that their moral evaluation of the actions of others would result in moral evaluation of themselves by others. Consequently, as a means of self-protection they judged no one's behavior as immoral, including their own. They are not unique in this. Parents today do this with their adult children who live a life-style contrary to all they were taught. Their hesitancy to make moral judgments may be due in part to the parent's reluctance to invite moral criticism of their own parenting. Teachers are hesitant to make moral judgments on public issues in bioethics (e.g., abortion), due in part to the fear of losing rapport with students and of being judged as being intolerant. Friends do this believing they will lose each other's friendship if they make a moral judgment on those who know them well enough to reciprocate with similar criticism of their own behavior. Of course these parents, teachers, and friends are right. They do risk return criticism. Adult children, students, and friends, like most people today, do not want to hear judgments made about their own behavior.

The rejection of the very idea of moral judgments is supported culturally by the notion that there are, in fact, no right or wrong actions anyway. It is widely accepted, at least in superficial principle, that morality is relative to the situation. This has become a convenient way of not having to wrestle with moral judgments in issues of bioethics today, choosing instead to champion the right of the individual to create his or her own morality.

THE ORIGINS OF SIN

But where shall we begin to face up to our lack of courage in the determination of what is moral and ethical? And how shall we know where to draw the line on what is morally good or evil, right or wrong? Long before doing so we need to look at some other issues. First, we need to look at the beginning of the Story God tells to see the origin of the problem. We need to know how we came to be the way we are. As people who live by the Story God tells, we begin with what God identifies as the problem of sin.

The Story actually begins not with the origin of sin, but with the origin of good. As Jesus said, "No one is good but God alone" (Luke 18:19). In the beginning, God made everything and everything was good. The first human beings were created good. Being created in the *image of God* as good is not the same as actually *being God,* and the Story reveals that our first parents wanted not only to be like God in being good, they wanted to be their own god and make the determination of what is good and evil. They challenged God for the destiny of their own lives. The Story unfolds:

The Lord God took the man and put him in the garden of Eden to till it and keep it. And the Lord God commanded the man, saying, "You may freely eat of every tree of the garden; but of the tree of the knowledge of good and evil you shall not eat, for in the day you eat of it you shall die." (Genesis 2:15–17)

The Story continues, as Adam and Eve are tempted to eat:

But the serpent said to the woman, "You will not die. For God knows that when you eat of it your eyes will be opened, and you will be like God, knowing good and evil." (Genesis 3:4–5)

Dietrich Bonhoeffer, writing on ethics, examines the problem as follows:

Man at his origin knows only one thing: God. ... [But] the knowledge of good and evil shows that he is no longer at one with this origin. ... But man cannot be rid of his origin. Instead of knowing himself in the origin of God, he must now know himself as an origin. He interprets himself according to his possibilities of being good or evil, and he therefore conceives himself to be the origin of good and evil. ... Man as the image of God draws his life from the origin of God, but the man who has become like God draws his life from his own origin.[1]

According to Bonhoeffer, the conclusion we must draw is that man has become *like* God, but *against* God. In the earliest account, the Story in Genesis 2–3, we see the source of the tension in today's discussion of moral issues in bioethics. Human beings are engaged over the question, Who shall be God—God or man? Who therefore shall distinguish good from evil—God or man?

SIN AND SINS

It is time to examine the meanings of the word *sin*. The word *sin* can be used in one of two ways. It can be used to describe the *human condition,* and it can be used to describe a *human action*. In the former we can speak of *Sin* with a capital letter as something larger than particular, individual sins, and in the latter we can speak of particular, individual *sins* such as adultery, theft, murder, and so on, the symptoms of Sin. When it is given any thought at all, the common understanding of sin today is not Sin, but sins.

It is crucial for understanding the uniqueness of a biblical ethic that we understand the distinction. Simply put, *Sin* is a condition whereas *sins* are the symptoms of that condition. Sin is the infection that affects all human beings, the faithful and the unfaithful alike. Sin is the condition of our alienation from God described in the Genesis account of events in the Garden of Eden. When Adam and Eve hid from God because of their nakedness, they were not being prudish but rather realizing that they were exposed as spiritually naked people.

The individual acts we commit called *sins* are but symptoms of *Sin,* our impoverished spiritual relationship with God. Whereas it is true that there needs to be what we might call *spiritual health rules* to control the outbreak of symptoms, the real solution lies in healing the infection itself. We need to have God make spiritually healing fig leaves for us to wear in this life as God did for Adam and Eve, covering their spiritual nakedness before Him.

The loss of the distinction between *Sin* and *sins* in our time has led to the trivialization of the meaning of sins. No longer are they viewed as signs of a far deeper corruption and sickness. In the trivializing of Sin, comedians joke about sins and television advertisers condescendingly describe their product as "sinfully delicious." The "sins" of our time, conveniently impersonal and safe to attack, are those social offenses of environmental pollution, racism, and homophobia.

In summary, an increasing reluctance exists on the part of many people to make moral judgments of any kind. We cited some personal reasons for this. We also traced the reluctance back to rebellion against God who is the judge of all. In rejecting God we also reject judgment. We saw that the Story reveals our problem to be one of Sin, and we identified *Sin* as a condition of alienation from God and *sins* as the sign or symptoms of that alienation. Understanding the meanings of sin is prerequisite for understanding the need for ethics as rules, principles or laws to set limits on the behavior of human beings. More importantly, understanding the meaning and depth of Sin reminds us that passing laws to prohibit unacceptable behavior, although necessary, does not ultimately get at the root of the problem.

NOTES

[1] *Ethics* (New York: MacMillan, 1955) pp. 17–18.

5

Law and Gospel Foundations for Ethics

LAW AND ETHICS

In God's continuing Story, it becomes clear that Jesus and the Pharisees did not see eye-to-eye on what we would call ethics. Appropriately biased as we Christians are in favoring Jesus rather than the Pharisees, it would be easy to dismiss the Pharisees as insincere and hypocritical. Indeed, Jesus Himself said as much of at least some of them. Paul the apostle, however, had been a very sincere, conscientious Pharisee before becoming a Christian. He testified:

> My manner of life from my youth, spent from the beginning among my own nation and at Jerusalem, is known by all the Jews. They have known for a long time, if they are willing to testify, that according to the strictest party of our religion I have lived as a Pharisee. (Acts 26:4–5)

Paul had devoted his life to paying scrupulous attention to the Law of God. Nevertheless, being a sincere and honest Pharisee, preoccupied with the Law, led to his undoing.

Dietrich Bonhoeffer wrote, "Man at his origin knows only one thing: God." He elaborated, "The knowledge of good and evil shows that he is no longer at one with this origin."[1] This means that since the Fall, human beings are no longer naturally devoted to God. There is a disunion with God. Devotion has shifted instead to the self and to a preoccupation with the distinction between good and evil, as if it were ours to explore and we were capable of handling the things that are of God. We are all by nature conscientious Pharisees in relation to God, and were it not for the victory of Christ over our sinful human nature, we would all be condemned as they were. Bonhoeffer continues:

> It is in Jesus' meeting with the Pharisees that the old and the new are most clearly contrasted. The correct understanding of this meeting is of the greatest significance for the understanding of the gospel as a whole. The Pharisee ... is the man to whom only the knowledge of good and evil has come to be of importance in his entire life; in other words, he is simply the man of disunion [with God]. For the Pharisee every moment of life becomes a situation of conflict in which he has to choose between good and evil.[2]

Because all human beings, like the Pharisees, are by nature out of touch with God until they come to faith in Jesus Christ, it is inevitable that human beings should mistakenly focus on the subject of morality as if it were the substance of the Christian faith. Even among those who have come to faith in Jesus Christ, there is always the temptation to slip back into preoccupation with morality and the Law as the key to our religion. And it is not insincere, although it is a mistake, that we should believe that the Law can enable us as sinful human beings to handle the distinction between good and evil well.

The message of many ethicists today seems to imply that the problems of good and evil can be dealt with through the mere application of rules or the freedom from them. The prophets warned of this trivialization, "Do and do, do and do, rule on rule, rule on rule, a little here, a little there" (Isaiah 28:10 NIV).

As sincere as we are as Christians, preoccupation with the Law, rather than the Gospel of Jesus Christ, will result in finding ourselves under the judgment of God together with the Pharisees of Jesus' day. The Pharisees did not acknowledge and pay attention to God's flesh and blood presence among them in Jesus Christ, the fulfillment of all for which the Law had been given. In point of fact, they held tighter to the Law and rejected him!

Let me not be misunderstood. Ethics is about Law,[3] but for Christians it is not exclusively about Law. In this chapter I will be critical of ethics based solely on Law, that is, on commandments, rules, and principles understood to be the means to our becoming a moral people. The probability is that the reader has never thought of ethics in any other way than as a matter of Law, as *rules to follow for being moral.* But as Luther said against Aristotle, we do *not* become good by doing good. Being a moral person does not begin with our behavior and the obedience to rules. It begins with the Gospel and what God has done. Ethics, then, for those who are in touch with their *origin* through faith in Jesus Christ, is built ultimately on the foundation of the Gospel, not on the Law.

THE USE OF THE LAW

Christians have always had the same difficulty as the Pharisees in keeping the Law in its place and not allowing it to obscure the Gospel. Let us define Law in this chapter and hold the definition of Gospel for the next. Paul, the former-Pharisee-turned-Christian, defines Law for us in a series of rhetorical questions:

> Why then the law? It was added because of transgressions, till the offspring should come to whom the promise had been made. ... Is the law then against the promises of God? Certainly not, ... the law was our custodian until Christ came, that we might be justified by

faith. But now that faith has come, we are no longer under a custodian. (Galatians 3:19, 21, 24–25)

The Law of God was given to His holy people as a fence or boundary beyond which people were not to go without defiling themselves before God. Christians have called this use of the Law a *curb*. The Commandments curb outward behavior, our symptomatic sins. The Commandments tell us where we may not go and what we may not do. The Law as curb is one of the legitimate ways we may understand ethics as setting limits to our understanding of good and evil. This use of the Law as a curb makes possible an orderly and outwardly moral society. The function of the Law as curb is applicable to Christians and non-Christians alike. The difference between the two is that the former seeks forgiveness when they violate the Law and the latter do not seek it. Even though people in a post-modern age may not acknowledge the Law as a curb because they reject all absolutes, most will accept the notion that behavior ought to be limited either by civil and criminal law or by the self-legislating autonomy of the individual. Such individualism is extremely subjective, yet it attempts to maintain an inner governance of human behavior. Even ethics committees in hospitals still follow the institutional rules as formulated policies and procedures, remnants in principle of God's Law. This use of the Law is the first step necessary in securing a society's orderly, continued existence.

Another use of the Law, particularly for those responsive to God's Word, is that of a *mirror* to show us our sin. We look at the Ten Commandments, for example, as a reflection of how we measure up to the obedience expected of us by God. And if we are honest with ourselves, we are often forced to admit that we have broken the spirit, if not the letter, of the Law and need to admit it to God in hope of His forgiveness. In the use of the Law either as curb or as mirror, the Law always accuses us of Sin. It tells us, because of sinful human nature, what the limits are and it shows us how we have violated them. The Law cannot declare us to be ethical or moral people; it always accuses.

There is a third use of the word Law that is more controversial among Christians. It seems to justify the use of the Law to address, not the limits God has set but the self-transformation of the person as person. By this way of thinking the Law can do more than merely control outward behavior; it can serve as guide to change the heart as well. If this is true, then it is hard to see why the Gospel is necessary, for the Gospel claims that unique function exclusively.

This third use of the Law is considered, by some, to be beneficial as a *guide* causing Christians to behave more as God expects of them. But the Law is not beneficial as a motive for change of behavior, and the use of the Law as a guide is deceptively misleading. In the use of the Law as guide, the Christian attempts to change his moral being through the guidance of the Law. This person claims to base his life on the Gospel for heaven, but turns back strictly to the Law as a guide for his daily Christian life here on earth. As we shall see in the next chapter, the Gospel is not confined to heaven; it applies and transforms us for life on earth as well. To revert to the Law, in this case as guide, can imply that all we really need is a little more guidance and added effort on our part to change man's sinful nature.

The Law as *guide* seems to be a kinder, gentler form of the Law as curb and mirror. The truth is that the difference between the Law and the Gospel is that the Law in any form fails to change the heart. The Gospel was given to do what the Law could not. "By grace ... not because of works, lest any man should boast," Paul warns those tempted to revert to living under Law rather than under Gospel (Ephesians 2:8–9). For Christians to be become preoccupied in their understanding of ethics as Law rather than focused on the Gospel of Jesus Christ is to repeat the disobedience of our first parents, to experiment with good and evil rather than to trust what God has done for us.

The chaos of Eden following the Fall is reflected by the moral chaos in which ethics finds itself today. Much of ethical inquiry throughout history is nothing more than a preoccupation with the distinction between good and evil. In this preoccupation human beings are always tempted to grasp from the hands of God the determination of what is good and what is evil. The *command* of God, "You shall not eat of the tree" was not enough to prevent it from happening. Nor is the Law as *commandments* sufficient. Law has become an idol in ethics. At best we may, with enough practice, live by Law and avoid certain symptomatic behaviors called sins, but we cannot avoid Sin itself. The Law is inadequate to address the heart, and the heart is where the sickness has taken its deadly hold on us. The Law is the MRI or CAT-scan that reveals the malignancy, but the Gospel is the cure that gives us back our lives.

THE GOSPEL AND ETHICS

The Gospel according to the evangelist Mark announces Jesus' arrival with the words, "The time is fulfilled, and the kingdom of God is at hand; repent and believe in the gospel" (1:15). Mark means believe the *good news* of God's presence in Jesus Christ, who has come to destroy the power of Sin and its dominion over us.

Jesus' coming had been anticipated from the beginning of the world when our first parents chose evil to supplement the good that God had given. In choosing evil, their own spiritual nakedness betrayed them and they hid from God. It was not their physical nakedness that led Adam and Eve to hide; it was their newly acquired sinful nature that led to their shame (Genesis 3:8). God confronted them and pronounced judgment. They discovered the consequence of Sin, "In the day that you eat of it [the tree] you will die" (Genesis 2:17). On that day death's momentum was set in motion for all of us. Because God is good, He immediately intervened with a promise. God pronounced judgment on the *serpent* (the incarnation of the Evil One), but He also announced Good News to mankind:

"I will put enmity between you and the woman, and between your seed and her seed; he shall bruise your head, and you shall bruise his heel." (Genesis 3:15)

Every word in this passage is significant. The *enmity,* or conflict, is God's battle with the Evil One. The first *you* referred to in this passage is the Evil One. The *woman* is Eve, but in the fulfillment of this passage it is Mary the mother of Jesus. The first reference to *seed* is all the followers of the Evil One. The reference to *her seed* is Jesus who will save mankind from the power of death. The crushed *head* is that of the Evil One. The *bruising of his heel* describes the wound of death that Jesus suffered while crushing the head of the Evil One through Jesus' death on the cross. It is this crushing of the Evil One that is the Gospel or Good News of Jesus' victory over Sin and death.

Between the days of Adam and Eve and the coming of Jesus Christ, God reaffirmed the promise made to Adam and Eve in many ways. God's promise of *seed* began to take on flesh and blood in the creation of a holy nation from whom Jesus would one day be born. The New Testament records:

In many and various ways God spoke of old to our fathers by the prophets; but in these last days he has spoken to us by a Son, whom he appointed heir of all things, through whom he also created the world. He reflects the glory of God and bears the very stamp of his nature. (Hebrews 1:1–2)

The unfolding of God's promise continued at the time of Moses. Earlier we noted that Moses asked of God to see God's glory, but it was refused him. The revelation of God's glory would have to wait until the coming of Christ, who "reflects the glory of God and bears the very stamp of his nature." In reply to Moses God showed, instead of His glory, His goodness. Goodness is revealed in the promise God made not to distance Himself from mankind because of Sin. God reached out to Moses and to all mankind in the promise: "I will be gracious to whom I will be gracious, and will show mercy on whom I will show mercy" (Exodus 33:19).

The *graciousness of God* may be understood simply as God's *undeserved goodness* toward sinful human beings. His *mercy* promised to His holy people through Moses is shown in His not laying on mankind the punitive consequences of Sin, namely eternal death. Instead, as promised, God took death on Himself through the death of His own Son, Jesus Christ.

It is hard for us in a postmodern, relativist age to understand why God couldn't simply wave Sin off and delete the consequence of death with the press of button, but that is because we fail to grasp the reality of God's Holiness and the defiling nature of Evil. The words Sin and Evil are not subjective value judgments made by God as we claim they are for us in this postmodern age. Sin and Evil cannot be blown off merely as God's divine *opinions* detached from their actual existence. Sin and Evil have a reality that had to be dealt with, and God made good on his promise to do so on the cross of Christ. The Gospel is the Good News, as Bonhoeffer reminds us, that God has freed us once again to know "only that one thing: God."[4] Evil has ultimately been taken out of the picture by God.

But the Evil One continues to limp along with his fatal wound until the end of time, when God separates his holy people from sin, death, and the devil forever. The Evil One is defeated. That may seem hard to believe, for we still see evidence of evil all around us. Yet the war is won. Inevitably there will be casualties in the sniper fire that remains, but of Christians it can be said that whether we live or we die, we are the Lord's (Romans 14:8). Those who believe the promise of God's victory in Christ find peace even in times of continued suffering, knowing that "in everything God works for good with those who love him, who are called according to his purpose" (Romans 8:28). Paul expresses the Christian's confidence:

> What then shall we say to this? If God is for us, who is against us? ... Who shall separate us from the love of Christ? Shall tribulation, or distress ... No, in all these

things we are more than conquerors through him who loved us. For I am sure that ... [nothing] in all creation will be able to separate us from the love of God in Christ Jesus our Lord. (Romans 8:31, 35, 37–39)

So now that we have this promise of God's victory, how are we to live ethically? As Christians we need not concern ourselves merely with what to do or not do. Rather, we keep our eyes on what God has done. Ethics for the Christian is primarily about Gospel, not primarily about Law, primarily about what God has done and continues to do, not primarily about what we do.

The Christian's ethic is to live by faith in Christ even as Christ lives in us. Our ethic is to repent daily and believe the Gospel. The promise is sure: through Baptism God makes us his holy people. In the Lord's Supper God feeds us with the holy food of heaven for life on earth. God's promise has been fulfilled—"I will be gracious to whom I will be gracious, and will show mercy on whom I will show mercy."

Ethics for Christians is not about what we do for God, but about what God has done on the cross and how that applies to us. It is the death of Jesus on the cross that transforms our lives, and it is the Holy Spirit who makes Jesus' death applicable for holy living. As Christians, then, we are holy people living holy lives.

LIVING HOLY BY FAITH

What shall we say then? Are we to continue in sin that grace may abound? By no means! How can we who died to sin still live in it? Do you not know that all of us who have been baptized into Christ Jesus were baptized into his death? We were buried with him therefore by baptism into death, so that as Christ was raised from the dead by the glory of the Father, we too might walk in newness of life. (Romans 6:1–4)

How does this new ethic work? Isn't there anything that we must do? Yes, "the righteous shall live by his faith"

(Habakkuk 2:4; Romans 1:17). Faith trusts in Jesus Christ when we are faced with ethical dilemmas. Faith is not passive, going with the flow as New Age passivity invites us to do. Faith faces and wrestles with the incongruities of living between the realities of what God as our *origin* intends and what life in a fallen world has become.

Living by faith is not easy. We do not hide from the pain and suffering of this world, erasing pain and suffering simply by erasing the people in whom we find it. It is difficult to live by faith, to see at times the problem so clearly and yet, perhaps, to do nothing but wait, letting God do or not do instead. It is more natural in a fallen world to grasp control away from the hands of God and take charge, trying to make things happen regardless of consequences. But that is the way of Adam and Eve's Sin, and ours. At times, faith requires our helplessness while we wait for God to act, but this helplessness is not passive. In our helplessness we pray and actively trust in God. At other times, faith requires direct action and we speak the truth of what it is that sinful human nature proposes against God. From the beginning and in the end it is faith that enables God's holy people to live holy lives.

In ethical dilemmas Christians must think, decide, and do good. We are still concerned with right and wrong, good and evil, for as Bonhoeffer says: "[There is] a judgment which is true activity of man, that is to say, a judging which springs from the achievement of union with the origin, Jesus Christ."[5]

The judging that comes from union with Jesus Christ is accomplished through the medium of faith. Faith is trust, but it is not trust disembodied from its source. Faith is a relationship. It is the relationship of trust we have in God. This relationship shapes our actions and decisions in day-to-day living. Laws, rules, and principles are signs of the relationship, but they are not the relationship itself; it is the relationship that changes the heart of the Christian and the core of who we are as human beings. It is Gospel, not Law, that ultimately makes us good or moral or ethical people in God's eyes.

Think of meaningful human relationships that have transformed your life. Earlier I described marriage as a primary transforming relationship. At the risk of thinking more highly of my own marriage than I ought, let me describe one way marriage has shaped my ethical behavior. As a pastor I have often counseled troubled wives. Looking back I realize how perilously close I came to putting myself in an awkward position with some of the women I counseled. That is, I could see how my supportive empathy could have been mistaken for an invitation to intimacy. Yet no invitation or intimacy ever developed, and I have now asked myself how I escaped this temptation. I now suspect that nothing illicit ever came of my counseling troubled women because I never communicated the message that it would be allowed to become such. This was never a major struggle for me because of my marriage. My faith-relationship with God and my trust-relationship with my wife filled my spiritual and human needs. I was never willing to break faith with my God or my wife.

I say all this with some awkwardness, since I do not want to imply that my marriage is some kind of Platonic ideal. Our marriage has worked because we worked at it daily. We end each day with prayer, confessing our sins to God before one another. Nothing piles up that endangers the marriage relationship, and by the grace of God our marriage has been blessed for over thirty years. Having a faith relationship with God shapes our lives and our behavior. It is no surprise to me that Paul speaks of marriage as mirroring our relationship with God.

Gospel Meanings for Ethics

An ethic based on Gospel reveals the Gospel meanings of our life together as Christians in relationship to God. The implications of a Gospel ethic for Christians extend to specific issues in bioethics. The issues that are raised in bioethics today touch on those primary concerns of humankind that have their key in relationship with God through faith in Jesus Christ.

The moral chaos we experience today is not merely due to the complexity of technology, but to the loss of a relationship with God that is revealed in the mystery Story God tells, the Bible. Having been seduced by postmodernism, many think that the old faith is not enough for today's problems. In fact, Christians do not lack what they need to resolve the conflicts in bioethics. What people may lack is a biblical perspective that re-shapes them at the core. We will surely need rules and civil or criminal laws to prevent sinful human nature from outwardly distorting what God has created. The ultimate solution, however, is not Law; rather, it is Gospel. The task of Christians is to know and live the Gospel in the face of the autonomy, relativism, and loss of meaning around us. We are challenged to witness to something better by how we live.

But Christians need help. We are not yet, and never will be in this life, a people who always live by faith. Even as Christians, the sinful side of human nature remains and resists the transformation of God's Holy Spirit. The war won by Christ continues to play itself out in us even though the outcome of victory is assured for those whose faith endures to the end.

We will briefly examine the nature of the opposing forces at work within the Christian, making it difficult to believe that we are, in fact, a holy people when we do unholy things. Law is not abolished for the Christian, but its function is narrow and earthly, not heaven-bound. Law for the Christian serves to accuse so that we rely on Christ. It continues to curb and mirror the sinful self, but it does not transform the Christian life at the core. That is the work of the Gospel.

SINNER AND SAINT SIMULTANEOUSLY

Christians may appear to others to be hypocrites. That is, it will always be evident to any critical observer that there is a difference, at least at times, between the confessed faith of the

Christian and the life a Christian lives. But the Christian is the first to point this out, and has a way of willingly doing so. Although a Christian may know the right, he or she does not always do it. It would be foolish and out of character for a Christian to claim that although he or she sins, he or she is at least better than others who are not Christians. While the cynic might accuse a Christian of feeling this way, no Christian could rightly claim this view. The apostle Paul, speaking to Christians in Rome, honestly admitted his frustration over being a Christian and not always acting like one:

> "I do not do what I want, but I do the very thing I hate. … I can will what is right, but I cannot do it. For I do not do the good I want, but the evil I do not want is what I do. … it is … sin which dwells within me." (Romans 7:15–20)

What Paul has identified in himself is a dualism in his nature as a Christian. Paul is, along with all Christians, *sinner and saint simultaneously.* What this means is that even as Christians sin, they are saints who are simultaneously forgiven by Christ. Does this mean we can do whatever we want because God will forgive? The key word here is "want." It is not what the Christian "wants" that is a problem, but what a Christian ends up doing that is sin. The Christian as saint wants to do the right thing, but finds that it cannot always be done. The reason, says Paul, is that "sin dwells within me." The Old Adam in us as an agent of the Evil One wars against the saint that God has created in us.

It is easy to become discouraged with the incongruity between what we intend to do and what we end up actually doing at times. The best repellent for discouragement and guilt is to speak back to the Old Adam in us with the reminder, "But Christ died for me and my sins are forgiven." The Christian need not become depressed or preoccupied with guilt; one continues to believe and rejoice in the victory of Christ over sin. The conflict between the Old Adam and the New Man in Christ will not go away until Christ returns and makes all things new on the Last Day. In Christ's return the saint finds hope, comfort, and joy.

G. K. Chesterton noted that the sinfulness of human nature is the only teaching of the Christian faith that can be proven empirically beyond a shadow of a doubt. It requires no great insight to demonstrate that Christians are sinners like everyone else, and it is not always outwardly evident that they are Christians at all. Even Christians must cling to faith in order to be convinced of their new status as holy people. No matter how conscientious they are, Christians continue to be sinners even while God calls them saints. Having said this, however, one would hope that there would be improvement of behavior in those areas of a Christian's life where there is a clear need for change.

The basis of sainthood is not behavior, but the forgiveness of sins. Because of Jesus Christ, the core of the Christian's life is no longer dominated by the power of Sin; we live by the grace of God's forgiveness daily. Christians are therefore, saints or *holy people.*[6] Realization of this paradox of the Christian as sinner and saint simultaneously ought to cancel the notion that we can reach outward perfection in this life. Christians who are continually discouraged with their *spiritual progress* have not learned to live with the sinner-saint paradox described by Paul and demonstrated in the lives of the faithful from Abraham, Isaac, Jacob, and Moses to all of God's holy people who ever lived.

The energy of the Christian life and the focus of holy living does not consist in trying harder to be good. It is humbling to have to admit to oneself that spiritual self-improvement is an impossibility. It may be pride, as much as conscientious desire for self-improvement, that causes us to refuse to believe our holiness is a gift of God in Christ, enjoyed and lived by faith, not by our own efforts. Faith requires us to entrust our lives to God, relying on the Holy Spirit to transform us. As our faith takes charge, we leave behind the narcissistic preoccupation with self-evaluation and put our spiritual energies into serving the needs of others.

As the Christian life is a matter of living by faith in the promises of God, so ethics for the Christian is a matter of living under God's grace in decision-making. Neither sincerity nor good intentions nor following ethical guidelines to the letter of the law will guarantee that our ethical decisions are pleasing to God. We can never be certain whether our thoughts, words or decisions are more influenced by the sinner in us than by the saint. Therefore Christians do not waste time in justifying decisions, but they live in humility through daily repentance. The Christian thinks, speaks, and acts in the confidence that the Holy Spirit is at work within and that sins are forgiven in Christ. The truth is that all a Christian can do is to examine critically the dilemma, evaluate it in the light of the Bible, and in good conscience make the choice believed to be consistent with the will of God.

Martin Luther advised similarly and suggested that Christians who are faced with the worst of ethical circumstances, where the choice is between the lesser of two evils, should *sin boldly* and *believe more boldly* still. Believing in the victory of Christ on the cross, the Christian is not paralyzed by indecision, but acts in faith, believing the forgiveness of sins that has been promised. To do so shows the boldness of confidence in the promises of God.

Trust in the gracious forgiveness of Christ does not treat ethical dilemmas in a cavalier or merely utilitarian way, nor does it say we are right merely because we did our best. Nevertheless, living in the forgiveness of sins frees us from the false notion that in a fallen world a Christian can make decisions without being influenced by the Old Adam still within him.

LAW AND GOSPEL FOR CHRISTIANS

This brings us to the question, "Does the Christian still need to live under the Law or is he now only under the Gospel?"

Is ethics for the Christian a matter of following laws or is it something deeper that transforms the inner person to think and act differently? The answer is based on the paradoxical nature of the Christian's life until Christ returns. Insofar as the Christian is a sinner he still needs to be guided by the Law, but in so far as he is a saint he is being transformed by the Gospel. We may ask, "How will I know which is operative when?" The answer is, "You won't." Therefore the Christian lives a life of daily repentance, honestly examining his life, confessing his known sins, and receiving the absolution God gives in Christ. Describing Luther's view, Paul Althaus concludes:

> In the ethical sense my action is good if done in response to God's command. In the metaethical sense my action is good, despite its constant impurity, because of God's act of justification.[7]

We attempt to do the good but know that sin infects everything and therefore we live a life of daily confession and absolution.

The function of the Law for the sinner-in-the-Christian is the same as that for the non-Christian. It serves to curb behavior that is wrong and mirrors the need for repentance when we see that we have done wrong. The Law, for Christians or non-Christians, always accuses. It never gets to the core of the problem and it never transforms the inner life, but we need it until Christ comes again and makes our whole being new.

The Gospel, on the other hand, makes its appeal to the believer, the saint, the new man within the Christian. The Gospel of Christ's victory over sin, death, and the devil frees us to live by faith in God's promise of forgiveness. The Gospel frees us to see the deeper implications of the issues in bioethics as an extension of the conflict between the God who enlightens our way and the powers of darkness that overshadow us, both present within us. The Gospel gives us truthful insight into the underlying issues. It opens up to the eyes of faith the deeper significance of Christ for our understanding of how to live in faithfulness until the end. Because of the sinful self that still resides within, the Christian needs the Law, but the Christian, because he or she is also saint, thrives on the Gospel as the only real good news there is in this world.

The second half of this book will examine the issues in the light of the Story God tells, the influences of the culture from which the issues arise, and the celebration of the Gospel which is ultimately the Christians ethic. It will become clear that I advocate no easy road for the Christian in ethical decision-making, as we examine the issues in bioethics one-by-one.

Although the reader might expect to examine issues at the beginning of life first and end of life second, we shall reverse the order. We shall first examine those issues confronting us at the end of life. By doing so we discover foundational meanings concerning biblical perspectives on suffering and death which also apply to many issues at the beginning of life.

Specifically, after a chapter on the meaning of suffering, we turn to those ethical decisions that confront us most often, such as the use of medical directives and the decision to withdraw or withhold treatment. We then move on to the issues of assisted suicide and euthanasia. Next, after a chapter on the meaning of marriage and conception, we examine those issues in what is referred to as *reproductive ethics*, including abortion, infanticide, in vitro fertilization, artificial insemination, and surrogate motherhood. Finally we conclude with those ethical issues that arouse our curiosity, such as genetic engineering and cloning, but which present us personally with little opportunity for decision-making at this time.

We shall view each issue from the perspective of the Gospel and its meaning for us as Christians. We shall ask, What are the implications of the Gospel in this issue for me as one of God's holy people who is both sinner and saint? In the end, as people living holy lives through our relationship with God in Christ, we shall find our wisdom and comfort in the promise of God's forgiveness and the transforming power of the Gospel. This will not get us off the hook in having to wrestle with difficult decisions, for there are no easy answers to some problems. The Gospel, however, does put the problems in a new light. We view them from the perspective of what God has done to give us a clearer vision of the world and where He is at work among us.

NOTES

[1] *Ethics*, p. 17.

[2] *Ethics*, p. 26–27

[3] The use of the word law here is not to be equated with civil law, but with the Law given on Mt. Sinai, including the Ten Commandments.

[4] *Ethics*, p 33.

[5] *Ethics*, p 33.

[6] The Greek word generally used in the New Testament to describe Christians is *hagioi,* translated "holy ones" or "saints."

[7] *The Ethics of Martin Luther* (Philadelphia: Fortress Press, 1965), p. 7.

6

The Meaning of Suffering

It is interesting that in this time in history when medical technology is capable of treating pain more effectively than in any previous generation, we should fear *suffering* more than ever. And we do fear suffering. We are obsessed with avoiding it at any cost.

Campaigns to legalize euthanasia in America readily appeal to our fear of the possibility of pain in illnesses we might contract in the future, even though most illnesses seldom lead to great pain and suffering. But alarmists propose that the way to deal with suffering is to eliminate it by eliminating the sufferer. They seemingly delight in raising such fears in order to motivate us to dismantle the Christian interpretation of suffering as something to be faced and accepted as part of life. They search out the extreme cases of suffering that serve as their text to overwhelm the general public and by it gain support for their liberalizing ethic which affirms the practice of assisted suicide and euthanasia. Irrational fears drive much of the popular machinery of medical ethics today.

As a hospital chaplain for over twenty years, I have seen patients tremble in anticipation of pain only to find that the ordeal they dreaded was not painful at all. This is not to say that medical procedures themselves are not uncomfortable or even exhausting at times, but not many can be called unbearably painful. Yet suffering, pain, and medical treatment seem to us inseparable. I continually heard from patients that it was not death they feared, but the suffering which preceded it, none of which, it turned out, they had experienced personally. Despite what we are led to believe by our fears, few dying patients suffer great physical pain that cannot be controlled. On the other hand, some pain is intensified or even created through worry and fear.

The topic of suffering in our time is complex and calls for definition. If, for example, what we fear is the physical pain of suffering, it can safely be said that pain due to physical causes is almost always controllable if proper medical knowledge and skill are employed. We can even visit pain clinics to treat the pain of patients who demonstrate no identifiable physical cause for their pain.

If by suffering we mean something other than physical pain, then we broaden the definition of suffering as a human experience. If we mean those fears, anxieties, and existential worries common to all people, enhanced by illness, then it may not be the physician who is most needed but a skilled and faithful pastor who sees as his ministry the *cure of souls*. The pastor's ministry to the suffering is founded on God's Story, in which the origin of suffering is traced to the Fall. God had said, "You may eat freely of every tree in the garden; but of the tree of the knowledge of good and evil you shall not eat, for in the day that you eat of it you shall die" (Genesis 2:17).

At the moment those words were ignored and disobedience followed, suffering entered the world and became a reminder to all human beings that we are sinful and mortal. Both suffering and death are the *fallout* of the human experiment with evil which God had warned us not to tackle. The good creation God had made became corrupted and anxiety was born: Adam and Eve hid from God.

A sense of impending disaster, free-floating anxiety, and loss of meaning in life are characteristics of postmodern times, even apart from serious illness and imminent death. When the normal postmodern dread is heightened by crisis of any kind, suffering becomes unbearable for many.

More often than not, people suffer and die the way they live. Only the Gospel can make it otherwise. In the rest of this chapter we will examine suffering from another perspective: that of our own experience and God's suffering in Jesus Christ. If we come to see suffering through the lens of the camera God gives us, we will take a different turn down the road than those who follow the culture of death, which in every way leads to a dead-end.

SUFFERING AND THE CROSS

Suffering is the result of Sin—not necessarily individual *sins,* but *Sin.*[1] Given the fallen nature of this world, some suffering is inevitable. In ethics Law and Gospel say different things about such suffering. The Law can only address suffering with the accusation of our fallenness, showing us our Sin; there is no comfort or transformation in accusation and judgment. Yet the world is never so bad a place that a Christian can't live in it. The Gospel is the good news that God has made of human suffering something other than we have known it to be up to now, both for our salvation and for our daily living. The Gospel is the transforming power that gives us hope in the midst of suffering.

Some time ago I wrote a description of one man's experience of suffering in an intensive care unit of a hospital.[2] At the time I was ministering to him as the hospital chaplain. It will serve here to tell this story as an introduction to the connection between the cross of Christ and our sufferings:

> Mr. Witti had asked for a visit from the hospital chaplain before surgery. Arriving at his room, I found him sitting in the chair beside his bed trembling at the thought of cardiac bypass surgery the next morning. A hardened man, not by temperament but by manual

labor, he said little but asked me to pray with him. We prayed that all would go smoothly.

That was nearly two months ago, and Mr. Witti is still a patient in our intensive care unit. He's alert, but he is respirator-dependent and requires dialysis several times a week. It might have seemed our prayer for a smooth recovery with no complications had gone awry.

What is remarkable about Mr. Witti, however, is his simple but enduring faith in God. Although he has not been able to speak for nearly two months because of the respirator, he asks me each day, through hand signals, to pray with him. I do. We daily ask for faith to trust God in all that comes that day. We also pray for healing according to God's will.

Each time we pray, Mr. Witti struggles to raise his hand to make the sign of the cross on his head and heart. As Mr. Witti knows well, Martin Luther himself urged us to do this each time we come before the Lord at the beginning of a new day. This sign of the cross is no perfunctory ritual for Mr. Witti. He knows, as Luther knew, that it's the "theology of the cross" that lies at the heart of one's confidence in the Lord.

Mr. Witti has a daughter. As we frequently stand together at the bedside, I often feel weary, frustrated, and empathetic toward Mr. Witti's suffering, but his daughter is all smiles and lighthearted, reassuring her father that all will be well and that God will heal him. "There's nothing to worry about," she says. But somehow her father doesn't seem comforted by this and turns to me to make the sign of the cross.

Unlike her father's "theology of the cross," Mr. Witti's daughter subscribes to a way of faith that Luther called the "theology of glory." She believes that her father will be healed because she believes that faith is the way to health, wealth, and success. There is no place for weakness and suffering in the will of God ...

Mr. Witti has surrendered to the will of God in confidence that God is on his side. Mr. Witti's daughter, meanwhile, is still trying to get God to surrender to her will for her father. In the theology of glory, we try to make God do what we want Him to do. In the theology of the cross, God offers to remake us in His image through faith in Jesus Christ.

The phrases *theology of the cross* and *theology of glory* are Martin Luther's phrases summarizing the inspired theology of Paul as distinguished from human ways in addressing suffering. Luther introduces the theology of the cross in his Heidelberg Disputation.[3]

> He deserves to be called a [Christian] who comprehends the visible and manifest things of God seen through suffering and the cross.... God can be found only in suffering and the cross.... Because men do not know the cross and hate it, they necessarily love the opposite, namely, wisdom, glory, power, and so on.

The way of God is to allow suffering to remain until the end of time. It is the inevitable sign of a fallen world. At the same time, God took on suffering Himself through the cross of His only begotten Son and transformed human suffering in fulfillment of the promise, "I will make all My goodness pass before you" (Exodus 33:19). The ways of mankind are to pretend that suffering is not suffering and ignore it, focusing on the distractions of human wisdom, personal glory, and the exercise of power.

Interestingly, much of the concern even on the part of those who do not claim faith is that personal glory and power have played too much of a role in medicine and bioethics. It is the way of our fallen human nature to continue the rebellion of Adam and Eve and to take charge of suffering in our own way rather than entrust all things to God. Such ways of fallen human nature eventually lead to death: suicide and euthanasia.

GOSPEL ETHICS AND SUFFERING

Assuming we don't simply ignore the sufferings of those around us, the first response to our own experience or the suffering of others is to attempt to do something about it. This is a natural, if not inadequate, response at times, just as hiding was natural but inadequate for Adam and Eve as their anxiety mounted in the face of the new experience called Sin. The *doing*, in their case, led them farther from the source of help and healing. And yet, it is good and right, within limits, to do something to relieve pain and suffering wherever possible. Christians are not sadists or masochists who enjoy pain and suffering. Compassionate responses to those who suffer are generated by the grace of God at work in even those who do not claim faith in God.

When we suffer illness, we seek medical help. When we are in the presence of the dying, we give comfort. But there is something deeply troubling about not recognizing how far we may go in rightfully addressing the relief of suffering. The Law, the Commandment, says, "Thou shalt not kill." In our anxiety to do something in the face of suffering, it is easy to dismiss what God has done about suffering. On the surface, we commonly recognize God as the ultimate giver of all medical knowledge, treatment, and technology for the relief of suffering in the sick and dying. We also recognize and turn to God in prayer for what He might do for us in the midst of suffering. But the Gospel is the good news that God has already done the greatest thing, far more important than providing the immediate relief we desire.

The Gospel ethic we live by as Christians is that in the midst our own weakness and helplessness in suffering, God is at work to comfort, strengthen, and be present to us. If suffering, as something more than physical pain, finds its source in the deeper anxiety we have about the apparent meaninglessness of suffering, then we should hear this meaning God has given to suffering in the cross of Christ.

The theology of the cross that comforted Mr. Witti comforts all who put their trust in Jesus Christ. God not only works through the suffering and death of His Son to reconcile us to Himself, but He also continues to work through our sufferings to sanctify us. When I am weak, God is strong. When I am dying, God gives eternal life. The cross is the paradigm of God's continuing to work in and through suffering in us today. As the place of judgment against Sin, the cross is also the place where God assures us of His love and provision in the midst of pain and suffering. Because Christ remakes us into holy people, we have the assurance of God's promise to be with us to bring good out of all we experience in this life. The working of good may not be evident to everyone. It may not be evident to anyone. But we live by a faith relationship with God, not by visual proofs and rational explanations. What matters is that God is with us and has conquered all. It was the experience of God's goodness, evident to Mr. Witti, but not to his daughter, that comforted him even as he knew he was dying. It was the Gospel relationship that transformed him from fear of suffering to being able to bear the experience of suffering.

There may be other ways that people find comfort in their suffering, but the Gospel is the way of truth that "calls the thing what it actually is."[4] Some may cope with suffering through detachment by means of techniques for meditation and stress relief, but these Band-Aid methods don't address the meaning of suffering. They bypass the meaning of what God has brought about on the cross. Techniques may offer temporary relief to those who suffer, but they fail to offer the ultimate good news. In the Gospel God has truthfully addressed what our postmodern worldview complains about as the meaninglessness of suffering.

Christ's death has given our suffering meaning and that meaning is Gospel to us:

> For it was fitting that he, for whom and by whom all
> things exist, in bringing many sons to glory, should
> make the pioneer of their salvation *perfect through suf-*

fering. For he who sanctifies and those who are sanctified [made holy] have all one origin [God]. (Hebrews 2:10–11)

In the days of his flesh, Jesus offered up prayers and supplications, with loud cries and tears, to him who was able to save him from death, and he was heard for his godly fear. Although he was a Son, he learned obedience through what he suffered; and being made perfect he became the source of eternal salvation to all that obey him. (Hebrews 5:7–9)

There is a joy in the Gospel ethic of what God has done for us that no other human activity can rival. The Law only accuses us of guilt and shame in the face of suffering, but the Gospel transforms the lives of those who are in Christ.

NOTES

[1] Sometimes suffering is a direct result of sins and not just Sin (e.g., a drunk driver causes an accident that results in his hospitalization and long-term disability).

[2] This article first appeared in *The Lutheran Witness* (July, 1989), p. 16.

[3] *Luther's Works,* Vol. 31: Career of the Reformer, Helmut T. Lehmann, ed. (Philadelphia: Muhlenberg Press, 1957), p. 52–54 passim.

[4] *LW,* Vol. 31, p. 53.

7

End-of-Life
Decision-Making

Grandma Richardson is sitting in front of the desk of the admitting supervisor at a nursing home. It has taken a long time to convince her that she can no longer live alone. Her adult children listen as the supervisor presents two documents identified as *medical directives:* a Living Will and a Durable Power-of-Attorney for Health Care. Such documents will determine, according to Grandma's wishes in the case of the Living Will and according to one of her designated children's wishes in the case of the Power-of-Attorney for Health Care, what treatment, if any, Grandma will receive when she becomes unable to decide for herself.

Hearing the word "will," Grandma agrees to leave everything to her children, but this is not that kind of Will. Her sons, assuming that the Power-of-Attorney means managing Grandma's financial affairs, agree to do so, but this kind of Power-of-Attorney has nothing to do with her money. In the Living Will Grandma is being asked to give the nursing home permission to withdraw or withhold treatment, even food and water, if, in their judgment, Grandma's treatment or care no longer seems advisable. In the Durable Power-of-Attorney she is designating someone she trusts to make that decision.

The Living Will made its appearance in the early 1970s. It was initially proposed as the first step toward legalizing euthanasia. It appealed to the fears of many that unnecessary treatment was often being imposed on unwilling patients. The Durable Power-of-Attorney for Health Care had its inception in Congress, in the early 1990s, motivated in large part by a desire to reduce health care costs.

Medical directives are presented as the patient's opportunity to exercise the right to self-determination in health care. Unfortunately, they have created an ethic that paves the way for assisted suicide and euthanasia. The terminally ill and the frail elderly are particularly at risk since, as the spin in the evening news repeatedly reminds us, this is where most of the health care dollars are spent today. It can be asked, however, "Where else would you expect to spend health care dollars other than on those who need the most care?" There is often a hint of resentment in such spending, since the terminally ill and elderly will not be around long to appreciate the benefits. The Christian's first priority is not economics.[1] It is the supportive care and treatment of the terminally ill and the frail elderly among us.

As we examine the Christian's use of medical directives, we acknowledge the legitimacy of its uses within limits. We also need to be aware of the issues that are symptomatic of its abuse. Legitimacy can be established by making certain the medical directive chosen will permit the dying to die comfortably, without either hastening or causing their death. But we need to confront some problems with medical directives. First, the use of medical directives has led to defining ethics for many as merely that which is legal. Second, medical directives can become a premeditated avoidance of the hard work of caring for the sick and frail. And third, the use of medical directives can easily deteriorate into a means of soothing our frustration over the general lack of control we experience in life events.

LEGAL VS. ETHICAL

Many are convinced that a medical directive, allowing self-determination even to the point of self-annihilation, is ethical simply because it is legal. Accompanying the philosophy of a medical directive, the evaluative phrase *quality of life* has become a criterion for determining whether to treat or not treat. The subjective quality of a life has become a criterion for justifying ending a life that some consider no longer worth living. The phrase *quality of life* is seldom defined and enjoys a liberal interpretation by both those defending a right to self-determination and those exercising power over the lives of loved ones. Much of the undefined nature of *quality of life* is what gives it power for the withholding or withdrawal of treatment that supports a frail life. The truth is that medical directives increasingly give virtual control over to, and serve primarily the interests of, those with vested interest in health care. Ironically, they do this under the banner of patient self-determination.

In the public arena, Christians could well work toward the modification of laws to restrict the scope and power of medical directives, and they should. But in one's own life, the Christian needs more than laws to shape his or her ethic. The good news is that God has given His saints more. The Gospel is the announcement that God did not defer to the Law which only curbs outward actions and inwardly only shows us our Sin. In sacrificial love God pursued our spiritual care on the cross. The Gospel will not leave Christians to live under Law alone but also proclaims the transforming power of the cross as the ethic by which the Christian lives and thrives.

SOOTHING AND AVOIDING OUR FRUSTRATIONS

It is unrealistic to believe that we can determine beforehand in what circumstances we ought to withhold or withdraw treatment. Protocols may be absolute, but protocol was made for the patient, not the patient for protocol.

The issue is not only that medical directives are unrealistic, but that they also tempt us to avoid wrestling with future hard decisions once a medical directive has been signed. It is easier for us, but more likely to generate abuse, if we defer to a prior agreement that is either too vague or too absolute.

The use of medical directives can deteriorate into merely appealing to our fears and frustrations over the lack of control we experience in illness. Patients, frightened by the publicity of horror stories in health care and their own bewilderment over technology in medicine, increasingly want to be in control of how and when they die. For some this means suicide or euthanasia. But let us not confuse suicide or euthanasia with the appropriate responsibility we bear for our own lives in the choices we must make in times of illness. The issue that is problematic is, however, something different than wholesome responsibility.

In stressful circumstances, both believers and people without faith in God can begin to doubt and become desperate; they may easily become obsessed with control over their own destiny. What else is there to do if faith is not present and active? This obsession has virtually become institutionalized in our health care policies. There is an increasingly desperate felt-need for self-determination and control among us. The medical directive can become an illusion that assures that in matters of life and death, control is ours.

In this obsession for control, Christians need to realize that being out of control is not the worst thing that could happen to us. The worst thing that could happen is to lose faith in God and grasp for control. Instead of being obsessed with control, we must entrust all to God's control. The Gospel is the wonderful message that chaos is conquered; death is defeated. We no longer have to fear either suffering or death, for the God who through His suffering Son brought death under control has all things under His control in our times of helplessness. Faith in Christ is the medicine that enables us to find comfort and contentment in times of trouble. Christ is our ethic that soothes, because He heals our fears.

WITHHOLDING AND WITHDRAWING TREATMENT

Perhaps the most heart-wrenching decision most of us will have to make at some point in life will be the decision to withhold or withdraw treatment from a loved one. There are surely times when this is appropriate. No one is required to receive treatment that is *futile* or which the patient considers *burdensome,* as Gilbert Meilaender has so well articulated. Some will say that a treatment is *futile* if it does not offer cure; but a treatment cannot be called *futile* that sustains the life, a patient's *God-given* life, even though we might all agree this is not the life anyone would choose for himself. Such may be those who are in a coma (persistent vegetative state) and receive food and water to live, or the demented Alzheimer's patient who needs to be tube fed because she can no longer feed herself or eat by mouth.[2] If the word *futility* is taken at face value as applying to treatment that offers little or no benefit, then such treatment may ethically be *withheld.* By contrast, it can only be *withdrawn* (having already been in place) if it does not cause death, for then such treatment could not be said to be *futile*, sustaining as it does the life the patient has been given by God to live.

As a criterion for withdrawal of treatment, Meilaender's understanding of what is *burdensome* is helpful. Treatment may be withdrawn, he says, if *the patient* considers the treatment to be burdensome. As subjective as this may be, the basis for this principle is that the burden of treatment ought not be worse than the burden of the illness itself (unless such burdensome treatment is transient and will soon lead to recovery). Nevertheless, Meilaender says that if the patient decides he can no longer bear a particular treatment and is not rejecting treatment *so that* he will die (even though death may come sooner rather than later), he is no longer required to bear the burden of the treatment.

Meilaender clearly believes that the determination of what is burdensome must be the decision of the patient and no one else. It is impossible, given the subjective nature of what it means to be overburdened, for anyone to say for another what is or is not burdensome. It follows, then, that the patient in a persistent vegetative state, or coma, cannot be said to be overburdened by the treatment of tube feeding or life support. Because a patient shows no evidence of pain or discomfort in a coma, treatment cannot be identified as burdensome.

Assuming such definitions of *futility* and/or *burdensomeness* are understood accordingly, there are yet other concerns problematic for Christians in withholding or withdrawing treatment. First, it is problematic when a patient's decision to withhold or withdraw treatment is motivated by an unwillingness to live the life God has given him to live. Lives limited by disability or illness lived faithfully are lives of worth because of the Gospel. Jesus' attention to the disabled and sick is a sign to us of the importance of the cross for the worth of all lives. The life we have been given by God in this fallen world may not be the life God originally intended us to have, but it is the life we are now called to live.

We may, in the course of the hardships of life, need to lay out our complaint before God, but because this is a fallen world we cannot make God the cause of suffering and death, even though He allows it to go on until Christ returns. God's delay in coming is part of the mystery of the Story God tells. The practical question is not, "Why has God allowed this?" but, "What has God done about suffering and death, and how can I now live with my own problems?" The great Story that gives answer to this is found at the foot of the cross. The lesser story of our own experiences may shake and confuse us at the moment, but as we are raised up by God in faith, there is also peace in the deeper mystery of God's love in the midst of suffering and death.

The second problem in decisions of withdrawal or with-holding of treatment may be an unwillingness to bear the bur-densome life of another. It is one thing to suffer personally and bear it; it's quite different to see a loved one suffer and be unwilling to bear it. But there is something wrong in reducing the question to whether or not we want to suffer. The only way to escape all suffering in this life is to die, but death is no friend with which to strike an agreement. Our peace and comfort as Christians is not found in how much or how little we may suf-fer, but in Him who suffered for us.

No one can determine for another how much suffering is too much. Only the patient, in the extremes of illness, can tell us what treatment is burdensome to him or her and what is not. What it comes down to is whether we are willing to accept God's Word, "Bear one another's burdens and so fulfill the law of Christ" (Galatians 6:2). No patient should be aban-doned to death for relief of our suffering. The Gospel is the Good News that God did not abandon us in our suffering but took on flesh and blood and entered into it with us. Because He bears our sufferings, we bear one another's with Christ. It is all of the same piece.

Laws, guidelines, or principles—if they are to guide us in ethical decision-making—must derive from a story that gives them coherence and meaning. In the Story God tells, the Law and derivative principles are guidelines for the Old Adam. They tell us what we must do and may not do; but they do not touch the heart or transform the inner person. It is the Gospel that motivates us. In the relationship of faith, and a sincere con-science that derives from it, definitions and decisions that result will not become manipulative ways of getting what we want. Daily confession and absolution keep us pointed in the direction of God's will.

God's forgiveness not only pardons our Sin and the sins of unethical decision-making, but it also cleanses the mind to live the mind of Christ. No Christian will make right decisions all the time, and when she does so for the wrong reasons she will still find her ethic in Christ who died and rose that we might be His own and live under Him in His kingdom, and serve Him in righteousness and innocence. In this we find peace, comfort, and the courage to live faithfully in the midst of suffering and death. The Gospel is the good news that in Christ's death and resurrection, our sufferings take on eternal significance for we are one with Him by grace, through faith.

DEATH

Death is not merely the end of life; it is the abrupt interruption of a relationship with God. Where that interruption is not repaired by God's grace, through faith in Jesus Christ, that interruption becomes final. It is called hell.[3] Such is the Story God tells. In Adam's Sin, death not only ends a life; it ends a relationship with God, body and soul. Severed from God, there is no earthly medicine to cure the dying that begins already when we are conceived and born and that eventually ends this bodily life. Being spiritually cut off from God, the soul loses all meaning and purpose in life. Without hope and meaning, we are left to breed and die as cattle. If this was all there were to life, it would seem that the most we could hope for without God is the distracted life of happiness found in a bovine existence according to the philosophy of eat, drink, and be merry, for tomorrow we die.

But this is not the whole Story. God has revealed a deeper mystery. In Adam death ended the life of union with our Creator, God, but in Christ we have been given new life that outlasts this earthly existence. Paradise is restored through faith in Jesus Christ! The great mystery Story concludes:

> Humble yourselves under the mighty hand of God, that in due time He may exalt you. Cast all your anxieties on Him, for he cares about you…. And after you have suffered a little while, the God of all grace, who has called you to his eternal glory in Christ, will himself restore, establish, and strengthen you. To him be the dominion forever and ever. Amen. (1 Peter 5:6–7, 10)

DEATH A FRIEND?

Before we can evaluate the appeal of assisted suicide and euthanasia as a response to suffering in our time, we must face up to the naïve belief that death can be whatever we make of it for ourselves. In our time we try to make death into a *friend.* In the modern scenario, death supposedly becomes a companion who helps us with our problem of suffering in this life. But death is not a friend. Death is an enemy to us and to God. In the end, death kills eternally.

This intrusion of death into God's Story was not something easily erased. Death's doomsday virus had corrupted the file of every human life and needed to be scanned on the cross before it could be deleted and God's program restored. Now, through the self-examination called confession of sins, we too must come face-to-face with death and discover in the cross of Christ the only hope there is, namely, the forgiveness of sins and the gift of eternal life. In Christ, because of Good Friday and Easter Sunday, death is now a conquered enemy. Yet death is still an enemy. We ought not make it a friend who helps us take our own life or the life of someone we love, as a response to suffering.

In these postmodern times the fear of death as felt by previous generations has taken a new turn. *Direct fear of death* has been replaced by the *indirect fear of death* called suffering. The fear of suffering is the postmodern expression of the fear of death and meaninglessness that comes with the threat of separation from God.

In the absence of God's Story, a human construct has been substituted for coping with the fear of death. It is the construct of a psychological interpretation of death. This interpretation does not concern itself with the spiritual meanings of death but proposes instead that comfort be found in an explanation of grief and the *stages of dying.* In an attempt to domesticate death and remove the fear of it once and for all, the stages of dying *(denial, bargaining, depression, anger, and accep-*

tance) are offered as an alternative to revelatory, spiritual meanings. But no explanation of the physical, mental, and emotional processes of dying can domesticate death's threat or provide the only real comfort there is. The Christian's comfort is finally that "if we have died with him, we shall also live with him" (2 Timothy 2:11).

THE APPEAL OF SUICIDE AND EUTHANASIA

The trend toward assisted suicide and euthanasia has become a way of coping with death as something over which people otherwise have no control. In the absence of faith in God, taking matters into a man's own hands seems to him to solve the frightening uncertainty of how and when he might experience death. It is a strange twist of irony that the fear of death should cause a person to seek it so deliberately and, in a strange way, eagerly.

Assisted suicide asks for more than death. It asks for public *approval* to kill oneself. Those who pleaded with Jack Kevorkian to end their lives could have, in most cases, done it without his help, but they wanted the sanction of official medical authority. The irony is that these patients are often angry with medical authorities, and yet they throw themselves into the hands of a medical authority that specializes in their self-destruction. Jack Kevorkian has never been involved in the care of patients. He is a pathologist, whose medical training is in the study of dead human tissue, examining the deceased by means of autopsy.

The excessive, indiscriminate killings, expressions of Kevorkian's obsession with death, have created a vision for the public not unlike that which is presented by a cult leader who demands a following to the death as the price of his acceptance. The choice of these candidates for death is predictable. Meilaender identifies the typical candidate presented to justify the argument for euthanasia as one for whom we might feel some empathy. He or she is one who would have died soon anyway, was suffering terrible pain, and asks to be killed, and appeals to the motive of mercy. The offer of death to such vulnerable and despairing people who have little control over their lives temporarily satisfies the hunger of Kevorkian's cadaverous insatiability.

Euthanasia differs from assisted suicide only on the technicality of who finally pushes the button. There is no moral difference between whether we kill ourselves or ask someone else to do it. God's Law always accuses: "Thou shalt not kill." The legalization of euthanasia in some locations in the country only serves to confuse ethics with legality, as if legal is ethical. However, those who live God's Story look to Christ and not to civil law as their ethic. The cross of Christ is the only instance of killing an innocent human being that can ever be called good, but it was God who made it good, not human beings.

AIMING TO KILL

At times, specific cases make the headlines in states that legally attempt to sanction the immoral practice of euthanasia. Most often, when practiced in a hospital or nursing home, euthanasia may not be so easily identified for what it is. Indeed, many nurses and doctors opposed to euthanasia might be unable and unwilling to identify their actions as sometimes constituting assisted suicide or euthanasia. Again, Meilaender provides some help in learning to recognize euthanasia when it occurs. He says simply that euthanasia takes place in the care of a patient whenever we *aim at death* as our goal.

> We must distinguish what we *aim* at from the *result* of the action. ... if we fail to distinguish between aim and result, we will be unable to see any difference between the self-sacrifice of a martyr and the suicide of a person weary with life. The result is the same for each: death. But the aim or purpose is quite different. Whereas the suicide aims at his death, the martyr aims at faithfulness to God. Both martyr and suicide recognize in

advance that the result of their choice and act will be death. But the martyr does not aim at death.[4]

Meilaender further warns us not to confuse aim with motive. He differentiates between the two, recognizing that some people believe they are not aiming at the death of the patient but at the relief of the patient's suffering. The implication is that compassion overrides ethics. It is clear, for example, that although the motive of a distraught father who disconnects the respirator from his son in order to relieve his son's suffering might indeed be motivated by love, he still aims at death to accomplish his goal. In fact, if he is honest with himself, his goal is the death of his child. If we believe, as God's Story tells, that it is wrong to kill the weak and helpless, then no argument for the relief of suffering, however well motivated by compassion, can make it right.

AIMING AT DEATH AND ALLOWING TO DIE

Meilaender describes the moral difference between euthanatizing a suffering person near death and simply letting such a person die. He writes:

> Suppose this patient were to stop breathing, we were to reject the possibilities of resuscitation, and then the person were suddenly to begin breathing again. Would we, simply because we had been willing to let this patient die, now proceed to smother him so that he would indeed die? Hardly. And the fact that we would not indicates that we did not aim at his death (in rejecting resuscitation), though his death could have been the result of what we did aim at (namely, proper care of him in his dying).[5]

Language is often used carelessly, and such is the case when people say that suffering people ought to be allowed to die. The problem is often that such suffering people are not dying and it is not a matter of allowing, but of causing, death. In reality, no one can keep a dying person from dying. But it is possible to neglect a suffering person long enough so that he dies. If a person is irretrievably dying, it is surely good care simply to be present with that person and in compassion keep him comfortable. It is also good care not to use death as the solution to his suffering. In providing care and not killing, we do what God does for us each day.

THE MALADY AND THE GOSPEL

At the root of the appeal of assisted suicide and euthanasia is the malady of our faithless response to the helplessness we experience with illness, disability, and aging. It is not the helplessness itself that is evil. Rather, it is the action of taking matters into our own hands and causing the death of an innocent human being:

> "Do you not know that you are God's temple and that God's Spirit dwells in you? If anyone destroys God's temple, God will destroy him. For God's temple is holy, and that temple you are. ... You are not your own; you were bought with a price. So glorify God in your body" (1 Corinthians 3:16–17, 6:19–20).

The assumption behind the desire to be in control of how we die is part of the myth that we are otherwise in control of life. The reality is that we have very little control over life at any time. Think of the countless aspects of life over which we have little or no control: our birth, parents and relatives, environment, our inherited mental and physical abilities, health and accidents, wars, the economy, opportunities (or lack thereof) for employment or advancement. Often the best we can do is make the most of our circumstances.

It is especially true that, as we stand before God in this life, we are helpless, finite, sinful creatures. Down deep we know this. Whether we are people who reject faith in God altogether or Christians struggling with the Old Adam, we hide from God as did Adam and Eve when we feel the helplessness of our exposure before God. The desire to grab for control of our life through euthanasia as a response to our helplessness is a defiant attempt to appear self-reliant when the truth is that we are totally dependent on God.

The Gospel addresses our Sin so that we Christians do not need to grasp at suicide or euthanasia. The Gospel is the good news that, although we are all helpless and without control over our lives before God, this is not bad. We need not fear either death or God. For God the Father has sent His Son Jesus Christ our Lord and fills us with His Holy Spirit so that whether we live or die we are the Lord's. He is the help and control we need and have received. It is a relief to know that we don't have to be in control of life. This comes as good news. We don't need to take matters into our own hands. God has taken matters into His own nail-imprinted hands and has freed us from the threat of death, the fear of judgment, and from hell itself. This good news of this Gospel transforms the life of the suffering and dying and brings hope and joy:

> Wretched man that I am! Who will deliver me from this body of death? Thanks be to God through Jesus Christ our Lord! (Romans 7:24–25)

The truth is that the Christian does not need assisted suicide or euthanasia as a solution to his problems. The Christian follows One who has overcome death and gives life. The Gospel of Jesus Christ is our ethic.

NOTES

[1] A recurrent myth in politics is that money saved in one place will be used well elsewhere.

[2] Although the Supreme court of the United States has determined that food and water are to be considered medical treatments because they are nourishment to life and not unique to the sick and dying, such nourishment ought always to be provided unless contra-indicated by medical circumstances (e.g., the inability to metabolize, organ failure, or imminent death). Food and water, however provided, are *not* in fact medical treatments; the legality of their removal does not constitute ethical decision-making.

[3] Someone has said that hell is God's permission granted to those who want nothing *more* to do with Him.

[4] Gilbert Meilaender, *The Limits of Love* (University Park: University of Pennsylvania Press, 1987), p. 82.

[5] *The Limits of Love,* p. 82.

8

Marriage and Conception

The aim of this book has been to explore the meanings of the Story God tells as they apply to the issues in bioethics that confront us today. The point has been made several times that truth and its meanings are not a virtual reality we create for ourselves but part of a worldview revealed by God and envisioning a heavenly reality. In this chapter we consider the heavenly reality that marriage has been created by God; it is not a social convenience created by man. As the earliest of God's creations, marriage was intended for the experience of intimacy and community in the lifelong union between a man and a woman. From this union comes the procreation of children.

In a fallen world with the decreasing capacity for lifelong commitments, divorce has become commonplace. With the growing number of dysfunctional families that sever us from past experience of healthier marriages, we are losing perspective on marriage as intended by God. With the growing number of divorced single parents, the not-interested-in-marriage women who nevertheless want children, and the intrusive presence of increasingly sanctioned homosexual marriages, the meanings of marriage, conception, and parenting as God intended them is no longer obvious to many. As Christians we are not called upon to redefine marriage to accommodate to cultural trends. Instead, God calls us to rediscover the meaning of marriage as He defines it.

In what follows it will not be so much our aim to address the meaning of marriage as a civil institution established by God as it will be to understand the meaning of marriage as a paradigm of the Christian's relationship with God and its implications for reproductive ethics. In this light the meaning of the Gospel as it relates to marriage will enable the Christian to understand what is at stake in the solutions proposed by reproductive technologies for resolving the problems of infertility. In order to proceed, we turn to the Story God tells. In the earliest chapters of the Old Testament He defines marriage:

> The LORD God said, "It is not good that the man should be alone; I will make him a helper fit for him." So out of the ground the LORD God formed every beast of the field and every bird of the air, and brought them to the man to see what he would call them; and whatever the man called every living creature, that was its name. The man gave names to all cattle, and to the birds of the air, and to every beast of the field; but for the man there was not found a helper fit for him. So the LORD God caused a deep sleep to fall upon the man, and while he slept took one of his ribs and closed up its place with flesh; and the rib which the LORD God had taken from the man he made into a woman and brought her to the man. Then the man said, "This at last is bone of my bones, and flesh of my flesh; she shall be called Woman, because she was taken out of Man. Therefore a man leaves his father and his mother and cleaves to his wife, and they become one flesh. And the man and his wife were both naked, and were not ashamed. (Genesis 2:18–25)

Another text, this one taken from the New Testament, provides us with the uniqueness of the Gospel meaning of marriage for Christians:

> Be subject to one another out of reverence for Christ. Wives, be subject to your husbands, as to the Lord. For the husband is the head of the wife as Christ is the head

of the church, his body, and is himself its Savior. As the church is subject to Christ, so let wives also be subject in everything to their husbands. Husbands, love your wives, as Christ loved the church and gave himself up for her, that He might sanctify her, having cleansed her by the washing of water with the word, that he might present the church to himself in splendor, without spot or wrinkle or any such thing, that she might be holy and without blemish. Even so husbands should love their wives as their own bodies. He who loves his wife loves himself. For no man ever hates his own flesh, but nourishes and cherishes it, as Christ does the church, because we are members of his body. "For this reason a man shall leave his father and mother and be joined to his wife, and the two shall become one." *This is a great mystery, and I take it to mean Christ and the church* [emphasis mine]. (Ephesians 5:21–32)

The Old Testament passage clearly defines marriage for all people, Christian or not. There is, in fact, nothing uniquely Christian about marriage per se. There is, however, according to the Gospel in this New Testament passage, something in marriage that only Christians can understand and appreciate by virtue of their faith in Jesus Christ. This is the hidden meaning of marriage that is the "great mystery" depicting Christ and His church.

THE MYSTERY OF MARRIAGE

If God's Story is a great mystery, marriage is, in part, a revelation of that mystery as it relates to husband and wife. Marriage is more than meets the eye. There a mystery beyond the promise of lifelong union with each other. The word *mystery* comes from the Greek New Testament word *mysterion*, translated in the Latin New Testament as *sacrament*. The meaning of the word mystery or sacrament suggests a visual *sign* of an unseen reality hiding beneath the surface of a thing. Marriage is such a mystery or sacrament, a *sign* of the nature of our relationship with God. Just as an icon in the Greek

Orthodox church is a picture that reveals the hidden presence of a deeper reality, so marriage is an icon that opens up the deeper meaning of our relationship with God in Christ. The submission of a wife to her husband is a *sign* of believers' submission to Christ. The submission of the wife to her husband does not imply subservience to domination.

In a sinful world, a wife's submission to her husband is sometimes occasioned by the fear of his rejection or by the threat of physical injury. Men who communicate such rejection or injury surely dishonor marriage and sin against God as well as their wives. Nevertheless, short of pathological endurance of abuse, when a Christian wife willingly submits to her husband she lives out of the paradigm of the church as the bride of Christ submitting willingly to Christ the groom.[1] The husband's unconditional love for his wife is the paradigm of Christ's unconditional love, which leads him to suffer on the cross for the salvation of all. Marriage, for the Christian, in its unconditional love and faithful devotion, has become the earthly enactment of the relationship between God and His holy people. There is in marriage, as St. Paul says, "a great mystery and I take it to mean Christ and the church."

The union of husband and wife in Christian marriage is an earthly sign of Christ's union with His holy people. In this sense marriage becomes a visible sign of Christ and His church on earth. In the Christian's marriage God teaches all people about Himself. As Christian wives are subject to their husbands and thus serve the Lord, so all mankind has a calling to serve God. As Christian husbands are devoted in love to their wives and to the Lord, so all mankind is called to love and be devoted to the Lord.

GENDER AND AUTONOMY

At this time in its history, contemporary American society is preoccupied with gender issues. This preoccupation arises from a prior preoccupation with autonomy. Concerns for autonomy are often expressed in terms of equality. Emphasis on equality between the sexes frequently envisions this in terms of a unisex sameness. Differences between the sexes are often de-emphasized.

If it really were true that men and women are the same, then it would be hard to justify the need for each other in marriage and procreation. It is, in part, in this American cultural fabrication that we find the promotion of a woman's right to procreate without a husband by means of an infertility specialist. In fact, if equality means sameness, homosexuality might be said to be the ideal and test tube-babies the goal.

God's Story provides quite a different meaning for the relationship between male and female in marriage. It reveals the meaning of this relationship in terms of complementarity rather than equality. Men and woman are of equal importance in God's Story, but they are not the same. Their complementary nature is created by God, not by human social arrangement. It is clear that they communicate, function, and relate differently. God created us as male and female for a reason. We have different callings or vocations to be who God has called us to be. We find our identity, in part, in the distinction God makes between the sexes.

The distinction is not one between a superior and an inferior being, for both male and female were created in the image of God. When God said, "Be fruitful and multiply, and fill the earth and subdue it; and have dominion over ... every living thing that moves upon the earth" (Genesis 1:28), God did not intend for spouse to have dominion over spouse. Their oneness prohibits it.

ONE FLESH

As it unfolds in Genesis 2, the Story describes the oneness unique to marriage in terms of a man and woman becoming *one flesh*. This *one flesh* meaning is a description of wholesome sexual desire, the man and woman looking upon the other as if the other were his or her missing half.

This *one flesh* union of the two expresses itself in the procreation of children. When children are not forthcoming due to infertility, this does not mean a loss of the *one flesh* significance of marriage. The *one flesh* significance expresses itself also in the unique intimacy and companionship of marriage as well as in the possibility of children. Children are a gift of God, but the gift is not given to all. This, too, is a hard truth for many to accept but implies no lack of God's love and favor toward a childless couple.

Because male and female were made for the oneness and companionship of marriage, it is not appropriate to think of husband and wife as autonomous persons contracting for equal rights. If, as is the case in our culture, individual freedom or autonomy is the primary justification for unlimited use of reproductive technologies, then it follows that marriage and reproduction begin to have little to do with one another. That is, if each person is free to engage in use of any and all reproductive technology available for producing a child, such as through the making of embryos in a laboratory and the implantation of those embryos in any woman, married or not, then marriage no longer has anything to do with human reproduction. The biological then becomes separated from the relational, and marriage no longer has the meaning intended by God.

It is possible, in a fallen world, to think of ourselves as being in charge of human life, of bringing children into existence by our own will when and how we please. Yet producing children artificially in a laboratory to fulfill a woman's right, to satisfy a researcher's morbid scientific curiosity, or to comply with a desperate couple's demand defiles God and the meaning of children as a gift from God to be given only in the fullness of time. If the command given by God to "have dominion" over living things does not apply to domination of spouse over spouse, neither does "subdue the earth" apply to the production of children in a laboratory without regard for marriage.

In an earlier chapter, I spoke of marriage as an illustration of the transforming power of relationship that shapes our ethical behavior. In this chapter we have seen how marriage is more than an illustration. It is a sign of the transforming power of God at work among His holy people to shape their lives according to His will. Marriage as the most intimate of human relationships between male and female is the paradigm of God's intimacy with us in Christ, shaping us to live as the new creatures we are in Christ. Marriage as the *one flesh* union of husband and wife is a reflection of our oneness with God in Christ, so that what we do to one another in marriage, we do to God.

ABORTION

To abort a child is to cause its death before birth. Infanticide is the killing of a child after it is born. In the debate over partial-birth abortion it has become difficult to distinguish between abortion and infanticide. In partial-birth abortion a third trimester living child is partially delivered through induced labor, feet first. While the legs, arms, and body of the child are drawn out, the head is permitted to emerge only partially. With face turned down the head is held partially inside the birth canal while an incision is made at the back of the head and the brain is suctioned out, killing the child. If the child had been permitted to emerge completely, the act would be indictable as an intentional homicide.

As hideous as this procedure sounds, the difference between partial-birth abortion and other abortions is only a matter of point in time during the pregnancy. In partial-birth abortion we simply visualize what we do in earlier abortions that we cannot see.

When abortion became legal in 1973 it emerged in a climate of concern for civil rights. At a time in our history as a nation when there was overwhelming support for civil liberties among minorities suffering segregation, the Supreme Court of the United States, influenced by the momentum, chose to make abortion a civil right. In so doing the Court repositioned the status of morality in discussions of public issues. Although the aim of the Court may have been to grant rights to pregnant women without making a moral judgment about abortion, the result was that the decision set a precedent for future life-issues that categorically excluded morality from consideration in public policy. Morality was relegated to the personal and private domain and disallowed in considerations of public policy.

This precedent set by the Supreme Court has created a paradigm for local public forums on issues in bioethics. Morality, formerly understood as being about objective or transcendent values of right and wrong, is no longer permitted as part of the argument. The word morality is currently undergoing redefinition. One ethicist defines morality this way: "Morality concerns, roughly, whether persons show proper regard for the interests of all parties affected by their actions and for any relevant rights, principles, or values."[2]

Note that there is no judgment of right or wrong. Morality is simply a matter of following the proper procedures and of not violating anyone's rights in the process. *Method* has replaced *content* in defining morality. It is in the context of this kind of thinking that discussions of the morality of abortion have been bogged down for nearly three decades in this country. Discussion of abortion always begins and ends with a discussion of rights: the rights of the woman vs. the rights of the unborn child. The ultimate morality of abortion will not be decided on the basis of rights; it will be decided on the basis of the Story God tells.

CREATED BY GOD

The point has previously been made that, following the sin of Adam and Eve, God made a promise regarding the "seed of the woman." A child, a son of Adam, would over-come sin and death and reconcile the human race to God. The promise of that child, the Messiah, was at the core of all hope until fulfilled in the birth of Jesus Christ. Until that time came, the hopes of God's people, including Eve as she gave birth to the first child, focused on each child born as the one promised by God.

It was not until Mary brought forth her firstborn son and wrapped Him in swaddling clothes and laid Him in a manger that the promise was fulfilled: "A virgin shall conceive and bear a child" (Matthew 1:23, Isaiah 7:14). From Eve to Mary, con-ception held promise and the hope of God's salvation for all people. Since Christ's coming into the world, the conception of a child, the pregnancy which carries a child, and the birth of a child itself have all been given significance by the One who was "born in the likeness of men" (Philippians 2:7). We who live since our Lord's birth, death, and resurrection have reason to see the conception and birth of every child as a sign and cel-ebration of how God once entered our world in Jesus Christ. We see every child as a sign of the Son of Man's flesh and blood presence among us. It is for this Gospel reason that the Christian faith opposes abortion on demand.

It has been said poetically, "Conception is the sixth day of creation continued in the womb." It might seem that a child created incestuously or through rape surely could not be creat-ed by the will of God. Indeed, the sin and violence that leads to such a conception is not the will of God; but life conceived is the will of God, for all life comes only from God however it is conceived in this fallen world.

It is not an unimportant observation in consideration of circumstances in which abortion might be acceptable, to acknowledge that pregnancy resulting from rape is rare. In fact, abortion for reasons of saving the life of the mother, or for incest or rape together, make up less than one percent of the million plus abortions performed in this country each year. It can be easily deduced therefore that ninety-nine percent of all abortions are performed for reasons as diverse as embarrassment over pregnancy, as a method of birth control, as a response to inconvenience, as a choice competing with financial obligations, as a preference for career, or as one way of coping with a stressful life situation. Although Christians may be sympathetic to women in some of these circumstances, the reality remains that a child's life is sacrificed for the sake of its mother where no threat to the mother's life exists.

Reasons for Abortion

It has been said that pregnancy resulting from rape is a continuation of the violence of such an act and abortion is therefore justifiable in such cases. It seems strange, however, that an innocent child, conceived during a rape, should be targeted as the enemy in a woman's understandable rage, as if the child were her assailant. The child is a victim of the rape much as is the mother. The child may be a reminder of the rape, but that is not the fault of the child.

Having counseled women who were considering abortion by reason of rape, it always concerned me that abortion was perceived as a solution to a problem, namely, a way of abolishing the living reminder of the rape. But a rape that happened has happened. It is real and has become a part of that woman's life. Rape is an act of violence against her that requires, among other things, supportive care and counseling. Abortion is also an act of violence adding self-inflicted insult to the experienced injury of a woman who has suffered rape. We might well be sympathetic to a woman who wants all reminders of the rape to be forgotten, but the reality is that both the rape and the pregnancy are real and can't be erased. For Christians, as difficult as it surely is, it is only when a woman, by God's grace, is able to forgive her assailant that she will also be free of the rage that threatens her relationships with other men, as well as the child possibly conceived within her.

The one circumstance most commonly accepted as a justification for abortion is a life-threatening pregnancy. The justification is simply that it is better, although tragic, to abort in order to save one life than to not abort and lose both mother and child. In a sanctified way, abortion under these circumstances may be an act of saving life rather than taking life, although no woman is under obligation to save her life rather than the child's where that is either possible or decided by her.

ABORTION AS A SPIRITUAL ISSUE

It is difficult even for Christians to think spiritually rather than emotionally about abortion, since the issue has become confused for most people through misguided rhetoric. Christians are the holy people of God and we defile God's holiness when abortion is chosen other than for reasons of saving the life of the mother. For the Christian, the question is not, "Under what other circumstances is abortion justified?" The real question for those who have chosen abortion is, "Where can I find a loving and gracious God who forgives my sin because I have chosen abortion?"

In a world where the choices are sometimes, but not always, between the lesser of two evils, even Christians will do wrong. When confronted by our sin, we are able to confess it and receive absolution. In order for us to remain honest with ourselves and with God, God has given pastors who serve in His place as they hear a Christian's confession and pronounce God's forgiveness. Jesus gave this power to forgive to the church, and the church exercises it through the office of the pastoral ministry. The forgiveness pronounced is as sure as God Himself speaking to us.

Those women who have had abortions need not make public their confession to the whole church, although their witness may serve to encourage others. But they do need to confess their sin to God. And God will forgive. Because of the weakness of human nature, a woman may need to return to her pastor from time to time to be reassured of God's forgiveness. Indeed, God does forgive. This is the Gospel that transforms the life of a woman who has had an abortion. This is the Christian woman's ethic: that Christ did through obedience on the cross what she did not do in obedience to God. His obedience has now been credited to her.

INFANTICIDE

Having observed that the distinction between abortion and infanticide is blurred in partial-birth abortion, the fact remains that there are other cases of infanticide, the direct killing of a newborn. The case of Baby Doe (Bloomington, Indiana 1982) was the occasion of Congressional action declaring infanticide illegal for reasons of handicap. More brutal cases have involved a parent who has simply chosen to kill an unwanted newborn rather than bear responsibility for its care. Clinical cases of newborns in a hospital setting have involved the birth of anecephalic infants (usually having only brainstem function which controls heart and breathing) and discussions of harvesting the infants organs before death which normally occurs within a matter of hours to days.

Although some might be sympathetic toward infanticide for an anecephalic infant rather than the brutal killing of an unwanted newborn by parents, the truth is that infanticide is, in all cases, the killing of a newborn child. Utilitarian reasons for doing so do not justify the immorality of such actions. Children are not our possessions to dispose of as we wish.

Infanticide involves the killing of the newly born because of the perceived need of the parent to resolve a dilemma other than through entrusting all to God. According to the Law of God, infanticide clearly falls under the commandment, "Thou shalt not kill." The word *kill* in this context is the killing of the innocent.

According to the Gospel that transforms our lives, the good news is that we do not need to resolve the dilemma by taking matters into our own hands, since Jesus Christ has taken the underlying matter of this fallen world into His own hands on the cross. We are not left to resolve life's dilemmas through sinful human actions. We find our ethic in the Gospel promise that "all things work together for good to them who love God" (Romans 8:28 KJV), even as they did with Christ and the cross. When decision-making takes place in the context of faithfulness to God's Story, killing is no longer an option.

NOTES

[1] Paul writes, "Be subject to one another out of reverence for Christ" (Ephesians 5:21).

[2] Kenneth D Alpern, ed., *The Ethics of Reproductive Technology* (New York: Oxford University Press, 1992), p 5.

9

Procreation

Reproductive technologies fall into two categories: those in which the natural parents are assisted in reproducing their own children, and those in which someone other than the husband and wife are personally involved in the process. In the former, sperm and egg originate with the married couple and the embryo formed is carried in the uterus of the wife. The circumstances are traditional, but the technologies assist. In the latter, the sperm and/or egg are donated by someone outside the marriage and the uterus bearing the child may be that of someone other than the wife. Techniques used in reproductive technologies may involve artificial insemination, in vitro fertilization, or surrogate motherhood.

ARTIFICIAL INSEMINATION

Artificial insemination consists in artificially introducing sperm into the uterus. This procedure is presently available in clinics to any married or unmarried woman. The sperm used may be that of the woman's husband or that of a donor. Sperm donors receive about one hundred dollars for their donation. There are presently no regulations regarding sperm donations. As it happens, in the past, donors have often tended to be medical students. The 1990s have seen approximately 30,000 births a year in the United States by means of artificial insemination among both married and unmarried women.[1]

Artificial insemination with spouse would seem to fall under the category of assisting nature and probably raises the least number of problems for Christians. The problem of collecting sperm is somewhat troublesome since the spouse's sperm may be obtained either through masturbation or through use of a condom in intercourse. Although disruptive of the intimacy of intercourse, collection following intercourse is probably more acceptable than masturbation, both because masturbation reflects a fallenness from what God intended for us sexually, and because masturbation has little to do with procreation, further separating the biological from the relational. When occurring between husband and wife, artificial insemination at least may not completely obliterate the one flesh meaning of marriage as some other reproductive technologies do.

The more questionable side of artificial insemination is that in which donor sperm and/or egg are used. The objection here is that donor sperm or egg obviously involves a third party in the conception of a child. For one thing, donation distances the biological from the relational, moving further away from begetting a child as a gift to the making of a child by the power of our own will. For another, since the one flesh union of marriage signifies that husband and wife become one, it is hard to reconcile the biological involvement of a donor without violating that oneness. In fact, the only way one can rationalize this as acceptable is to disavow the connection between the biological and the relational and abandon the biblical meaning of procreation.

IN VITRO FERTILIZATION

In vitro (Latin for *in glass*) fertilization consists in uniting sperm and egg outside the uterus, in a laboratory, in a petri dish. The first "test tube" baby born of this method was Louise Brown, in England, in 1978. In the ten years that followed, approximately 3,500 births per year were achieved by in vitro fertilization.[2]

With in vitro, a woman seeking pregnancy experiences an expensive ordeal. She is required to submit to repeated attempts at implantation every few months, for sometimes up to a year, until conception is either proven successful or, due to failure to achieve pregnancy, she abandons the process altogether. Most often a pregnancy is not achieved since only 15 to 20 percent of couples are successful. The cost to a couple for in vitro fertilization is in the neighborhood of $25,000, a considerable sum for most couples, whether successful or not, and is not usually covered by medical insurance. There is sometimes a need for counseling for those who are among the disappointed eighty to eighty-five percent who must face their own inability to conceive and begin to think of themselves as "failures." Perhaps there is also a need for spiritual counsel among those believe they have "achieved success" by their own hand and not by the grace of God. Even Christian couples who want to live faithfully often have little understanding of the meaning of what they do, living as we all do in an age that justifies choices on the basis of good intentions and feelings, rather than on biblical meanings and the objectivity of the Word of truth.

With in vitro fertilization, couples endure a process that raises them up and slams them down as each attempt fails to achieve a pregnancy. The process is a complicated one for the woman and demands endurance. The ovaries are stimulated to produce more eggs than normal and several eggs are harvested at a time. Since each attempt at the retrieval of eggs involves some risk to the woman, more eggs are harvested than needed in the event multiple attempts have to be made to achieve pregnancy. When an embryo has formed in vitro, after a few days, it is placed inside the uterus of the recipient in hopes of the embryo implanting itself. The embryo may or may not implant and several attempts may be made over a period of months.

An embryo may be formed by means of in vitro under any one of a number of conditions. The sperm and egg that are artificially united may be that of the husband and wife. The sperm or egg or both may be from donors. Moreover, the woman who will receive the resulting embryo for implantation may or not be the biological mother. Finally, because of the low success rate for achieving pregnancy, several embryos are created at one time and stored for repeated attempts. Embryos which are not used are eventually either destroyed or used for experimentation in research, neither of which are options acceptable from a Judeo-Christian perspective.

It has recently been suggested, by no less a source than the Vatican, that leftover embryos might well be given up for adoption rather than be destroyed or used for research. But as good a solution as this may appear to be, it raises several new problems. First, whenever such social transactions occur in a free-market economy as ours, an industry seems to arise. In the case of reproductive technology, the very problem we seek to avoid is encouraged. Second, children as embryos could tend to be treated more as commodities than as human beings just as the fetus is already referred to in abortion clinics as a "product of conception." Third, it is difficult for parents not to think of their stored embryos as possessions banked for the future, further commodifying children. Court battles over the ownership of stored embryos attest to this. Fourth, it seems to be true that what we as society permit we also encourage. If adoption of embryos were to become a trendy norm, particularly among a sub-cultural elite which already despises marriage, in vitro fertilization itself might become normative, being justified on the grounds of it being for a good cause, namely to help childless couples. Fifth, the adoption of embryos for implantation by strangers might add to the as yet unknown risk of producing a new generation of persons who are no longer capable of seeing any need for or connection between the biological and the relational in marriage and conception.

SURROGATE MOTHERHOOD

In surrogate motherhood, also referred to in our euphemistically friendly culture as *collaborative reproduction,* a child is carried to full-term in the uterus of a woman other than the child's biological mother, most often for a fee of somewhere around $10,000. The number of surrogate arrangements is difficult to ascertain, but it is estimated that thousands of children are born as a result of this method each year. Pregnancy in the case of a surrogate mother may be achieved in any number of combinations, making use of the sperm and/or egg of the married couple, the surrogate's own egg, or sperm and/or egg of a donor.

There are problems with surrogate motherhood when measured over against a biblical perspective. The same objection may be made regarding the violation of the one flesh union as is true with donor sperm or egg. But, as Gilbert Meilaender points out, the most disturbing thing about surrogacy is that there is something amiss in creating a child for the express purpose of giving it away, where bonding is a planned denial before conception even takes place. This creates social and psychological problems for both surrogate mother and child. Numerous court battles, in which the surrogate mother changes her mind and wants to keep the child, attest to this sad reality.

We must never forget that children are a gift from God. They are not commodities to be bargained for and sold off, as is the case when a surrogate mother negotiates a price for her services. It seems disturbingly close to something like prostitution when a woman sells the use of her body for surrogacy. In those cases where a woman offers to bear the child of a friend or relative without exchange of money, there remains the objection that children are to be the gift that comes by means of our love-making in marriage, and not a possession to be bargained over even at the cost of friendship or good intentions.

Surrogacy is not the same as traditional adoptive procedures. In adoption a child is not conceived for the purpose of giving it away. Unlike surrogacy, which violates the one-flesh meaning of marriage, in adopting a child the prospective parents are enacting the biblical practice of welcoming an existing homeless stranger into their midst. Unplanned children are cared for in adoption. In surrogacy, intentionally planned children are sold or given away in the same manner we sell or give away commodities.

A number of cases illustrate the tragedy of surrogacy, when procreation is turned into reproduction. In California, a case was presented in court in which eight people claimed to be the mother and father of a child. An infertile couple had negotiated with a woman (who was also married) to serve as surrogate, while also contracting with a sperm donor (married) and an egg donor (married) to produce an embryo by means of in vitro fertilization. When the child was born all claimed the child as theirs. In a precedent-setting court battle the judge ruled that since there were no laws to govern this kind of case, the child had no parents. One wonders what this means to this child as it grows up without lineage or identity and what this does to a society populated by such disconnected and potentially dysfunctional people.

REPRODUCTION VS. PROCREATION

As difficult as it may be to create technologies capable of bringing together sperm and egg under rare circumstances and thereby producing a child, it is even more difficult to grasp the meaning of what we are doing in taking charge of this sacred domain of human life. Because it is difficult to determine objectively the meaning of reproductive technologies and because people do not want to be hindered in their quest for a child, they tend to ignore the meaning of what they are doing.

They become defensive regarding the use of such technologies. To put it simply, we want what we want, whatever it takes. That in itself shifts the focus from receiving a child as a gift of God to demanding a child made with our own hands.

One way to begin to unveil the meaning of what we do is to look at the language we use to describe it. The language of "producing a child" or the words *reproduction* and *reproductive technologies* betray a metaphor with a meaning all its own. It is the language of industry and the making of products. The image of commodities, the factory production line and quality control, the rejection of inferior products that do not measure up to specifications—all this comes to mind in the presence of reproductive technologies.

Once we have accepted the language, we also accept the concepts that accompany it. Hence, amniocentesis and ultrasound during pregnancy lead to our acceptance or rejection of what clinicians now refer to as the "product of conception." The aim of pregnancy screening is quality control. Abortion is the rejection of the product when it is found to be inferior or disappointing. In the end, the word *reproduction,* as making or manufacturing a product, brings with it a meaning that shapes our entire understanding of who we are and what we do. This language of reproduction is a distant cry from the meaning of the language of procreation which arises from the Bible.

The meaning of the word *procreation* is expressed in older translations of the Bible as the word *beget.* In begetting, life comes into being as the outcome of a husband and wife's love for each other. Procreation is not the aim of their love but the result of it. The aim of love is to love. Love is not utilitarian and has no aim other than to express itself to another. In loving, a husband and wife beget children and what they beget is like themselves.

In contrast to that, the meaning of the word reproduction implies a primary aim of making something for our use. Although we may speak of making a baby through normal intercourse, the truth is that we have little control over what is being made. In other uses of the word *make* we set out to put it together with our own hands. What we normally *make* is something other than a human life. When we make something, we seldom think of it as coming into being as the result of love but rather as the result of skill and our need.

We *beget* children because they result from our lovemaking. We *make* tables, clothes, and computers because we need them for our physical or psychological use. It may be objected that men and women pursuing parenthood through reproductive technologies do not speak or even think in terms of these distinctions, but that is precisely the point. We need to ask about the meaning of what it is we are really doing when we make use of reproductive technologies.

Having a child can mean many things to us. Ethicist Kenneth Alpern lists reasons having children: the expectation of a cultural norm; the symbol of the significance of our marriage; children are rewarding and fulfilling; a way of continuing oneself or one's family line; for the experience of pregnancy itself; a way of recapturing one's own youth; for our emotional support.[3] As much as every parent's desire for children carries with it the burden of a parent's needs or expectations, such baggage for the child is heightened for the child conceived by reproductive technologies. Seldom is serious consideration given to the good of the child conceived by these means. One feminist even argues that to ask what is best for the child with regard to the use of reproductive technologies is to undermine the right of a woman to abort by asking her the question, "What is best for the child within me?"

ONE FLESH AND PROCREATION

The relationship of marriage is a *one flesh* union of husband and wife, described as such in Genesis 2 and confirmed in Ephesians 5. In reproductive technology the biological becomes separated from the relational. The one flesh union is frequently violated.

While the mystery of the one flesh union of marriage has implications for many aspects of life together as husband and wife, it has especially profound meaning for matters involving reproductive technologies. A one flesh union, by its very definition, involves two people who become one in marriage. The introduction of a third person into the marriage through contribution as donor of sperm or egg, or through surrogacy, violates the one flesh union of marriage.

The use of a donor defiles the holy estate of marriage. The introduction of a third person in the conception of a child is, in essence, adulterous. We may think of adultery as involving lust and illicit sexual desire and conclude that none of this is present in the contribution made by, or accepted from, donors. To interpret adultery in these postmodern, psychological terms is to empty the objective meaning of the biblical prohibition against adultery. The meaning of adultery can be heard clearly in the Old Testament prophetic voices that issued warnings against Israel's adulterous worship of other gods. Adultery at the root is a divided loyalty, a defiling of our oneness in marriage and, at the same time, our oneness with God.

Whether understood as the passion normatively associated with adulterous behavior or the passionate desire for a child, adultery is ultimately the unwillingness to face up to and accept the life God has given us. It is that life which deserves our attention and not the life to which we are not entitled. It is the demand for what God has not given and the taking of matters into our own hands through the illicit involvement of a third person that are at stake in the use of donor sperm or egg and surrogacy. The fact that this adulterous action is performed antiseptically and in a laboratory does not negate the meaning of what it is that we do. What we do is to violate the one flesh meaning of marriage according to the Story God tells.

The one flesh meaning of marriage is also hindered when the *intimacy of marriage* is sacrificed through reproductive technologies. In vitro fertilization means that no physical contact between husband and wife is required. The child does not come into being as a result of our lovemaking but as a result of a technician's skill. This is not to say that husband and wife cannot continue to love each other and express intimacy at other times, although most reports by couples making use of technologies indicate much strain on the marriage during this process. But it is to say that the one flesh meaning of marriage is objectively absent in that most significant moment in a couple's life.

In surrogate motherhood, not only is the one flesh union violated, but so is the significance of the mother and child relationship. In surrogacy a child is specifically created for the purpose of giving it away. Bonding between mother and child is, of necessity, denied. The gift God gives is rejected by the one who carried that gift for nine months.

There may be some reproductive technologies that do not violate the one flesh union of marriage such as artificial insemination between husband and wife or the use of fertility drugs to enhance ovulation or viability of the husband's sperm. Yet the danger in reproductive technologies is always that conception takes on a higher priority than the marriage itself. The one flesh union is perilously jeopardized under the strain and demands we make upon ourselves, on each other, and on God. Couples do well to ask concerning reproductive technologies, What does this mean for the one flesh union of our marriage and for our relationship with God?

THE GOSPEL AND REPRODUCTIVE ETHICS

The uses of donor sperm and egg and surrogate motherhood and the conception of children outside of marriage draw criticism from the Scriptures. In addition to the violation of the one flesh union of marriage, there is also an unholiness in the *demand* for a child as opposed to the passive, but joyful, reception of a child as a gift from God. There is an exhausting weariness and desperation that grows with each failed attempt at pregnancy by reproductive technology. That desperation often turns into bitterness and blaming between husband and wife.

When no child results after months and years of money spent and failed efforts, depression or divorce frequently follows. Everything in life has focused on producing a child. The marriage relationship, where lovemaking is burdened with the weight of reproductive technology rather than with unhindered love for each other, may have become secondary, while the arrival of a child is expected to set all things right again.

No human being, especially our children, should have to bear all the burden of meeting our needs. Our deepest needs can only be met by God and the only human being to whom we can turn in our desperation is the God-become-Man, Jesus Christ. Only the Gospel of Jesus Christ can transform the desires of a childless couple for fulfillment-through-a-child into the desire for one Child born in Bethlehem. He alone can give meaning and fulfillment to our lives.

A final word needs to be said regarding those children who are conceived and born with the use of reproductive technology. Children born of such, even those conceived by donors or through surrogacy, are no less the children God Himself created. This is not to say that the end justifies the means and that all we have said is negligible. The fact that our sinful nature is at work in assisted reproduction does not lessen the truth that all life comes from God, however conceived. The child born of five parents (sperm donor, egg donor, surrogate mother, and two legal parents) will bear an additional burden in life growing up wondering who and whose he is. The identity crisis of teen years together with a confused lineage will not make life easier for a child, but the certainty of who and Whose we all are is found in Holy Baptism where God longs to make each child His own. This is the grace of God that accompanies life in a fallen world.

NOTES

[1] Lawrence J. Kaplan and Carolyn M. Kaplan, "Natural Reproduction and Reproduction-Aiding Technology," in *The Ethics of Reproductive Technology*, p. 24.

[2] Ibid., p. 26.

[3] "Genetic Puzzles and Stork Stories: On The Meaning and Significance of Having Children," in *The Ethics of Reproductive Technology*, p. 151.

10

Genetic Engineering

Would it not be a good thing to determine a person's genetic predisposition to particular diseases and eliminate those diseases long before symptoms even appear? This, in principle, is the most persuasive argument for genetic engineering and gene therapy.

Genes are the carriers of our predisposition for future illnesses. Genes also give us those specific traits that identify us as unique individuals. It has never been possible to change some of what we inherit, like eye color, whereas some of what we inherit has been changeable through diet, habits in lifestyle, and environment. The new possibility on the horizon of genetic engineering is that of altering individual genes so that all traits, whether eye color or illness, can be controlled. In theory, even parents who want to design their own unborn children, giving them traits valued by the parents or by society will be able to do so. Genetically inherited disease and unwanted traits will, in theory, be eliminated.

These are the aims of genetic engineering. Whether they can be accomplished or not remains to be seen. The curiosity aroused in us and the temptation to pursue such science fiction goals must be tempered with caution. Life itself and the human body are far more complex than we realize.

A more pressing concern has to do more with the world-view and beliefs that feed the frenzy of such thinking. Are the attitudes and aims which drive our curiosity about these possibilities compatible with the Story God tells about the meaning of life? Or are we merely Adam and Eve again taking the first step away from God by considering whether the forbidden fruit is tasty or not?

GENOMES, EUGENICS, AND GENOCIDE

The total number of genes in a human being is called the human *genome* (pronounced gee-nome). Funded by the federal government, the Human Genome Project has identified and mapped out the function of each gene with the hope that geneticists will then be able to manipulate genes to accomplish the aims of genetic engineering.

One of the aims of geneticists is called *eugenics*. Eugenics is the selective enhancement of certain characteristics or traits in certain human beings. Eugenics is not new, but the technology of genetic engineering to accomplish it is new. Eugenics has been with us since the beginning of man's conflict with man, for eugenics has historically taken the form of what we have come to know as racial and ethnic cleansing. Eugenics in the past has been clearly recognized in the practice of *genocide:* the wholesale extermination of peoples, and the practice of voluntary and involuntary sterilization, along with voluntary and involuntary selective breeding. Whole nations, and minorities of "undesirable" peoples within nations, have been scheduled for extinction. This is evident in the twentieth century accounts of the Armenian massacres in Turkey, the Holocaust in Germany, the bloodshed of Cambodia, the racial wars of the Balkans, and the tribal warfare of African nations.

The new eugenics offers a deceptively kinder, gentler form of bringing about such politically motivated changes. Because there appears to be little overt violence or coercion in the new eugenics, and because it does not seem to target any one group of people, many people will find the new eugenics appealing. But it must be remembered that past violence has only been the means, not the aim, of eugenics. Even when the violence is eliminated, the aim of eugenics remains the same. Eugenics still aims at valuing certain persons over others, and it views certain people as being desirable and others undesirable.

Even without violence or compulsion, eugenics sends the message of what is acceptable in a human being and what is not. Ultimately, it is implied that some people and their traits should and must be eliminated for the good of the human race. The means are at hand to accomplish this, and if the aberrant, dysfunctional lives paraded before us on TV talk shows do not show us who might be vulnerable to the temptation of the new eugenics, nothing will.

If eugenics is practiced, who shall determine what that uniformity will be and who shall control it? It matters little whether the individual or society as a democratic entity makes the choice, for the end result is the same: genocide. Value placed on the myth of autonomy, in which it is said that each person must decide for himself what is right for him or her, will no doubt be employed in defense of eugenics. But autonomy is relative to the ideologies and philosophies that shape it. Freedom to choose is not enough when the choice ends in the elimination of human lives counted as dispensable. Unfortunately we have already experienced this in the genocide of abortion. The new culture wars between those who live by God's Story and those who live by the myth of autonomy may be fought in the future on the battleground of eugenics and genetic engineering.

HEALING DISEASE

Having been as critical as I have been regarding the implications of genetic engineering, I must admit some sympathy for gene therapy, which aims to heal disease rather than to enhance human traits. Jesus healed the sick. The apostles did the same. In the gospel accounts, healing was a sign of the presence of the kingdom of God and of the Gospel itself.

The offer of healing through gene therapy needs to be examined critically, lest we harm more than heal. For example, discovering an individual's genetic predisposition for an illness for which there is no cure can only increase that person's anxiety and possibly pose the temptation of suicide. Similar attempts to alter the course of disease through gene therapy may disturb other genetically controlled mechanisms creating new problems for humans. In theory at least, we might favor gene therapy for the aim of healing disease much as we do with the use of other technologies. It is not technology itself that is harmful or wrong, but the misuse that derives from it.

Genetic changes can be made in two kinds of cells in the human body, somatic cells and germline cells. I will not spend a great deal of time in making a distinction between *somatic* cell and *germline* cell therapy except to say that the former (somatic cells) affects only my own body and the latter (germline) affects that which I pass on to my children. Some ethicists have raised concerns about the legitimacy of altering our own genetic makeup as compared with altering that of our as yet unborn children. The questions ethicists raise regarding these matters is usually confined to concerns for autonomy, civil rights, and issues of informed consent.

Our concern is more foundational to the whole question of what it means to be designed by God and not by man. Our concern has to do with the meanings of what we do according to God's Word. Our concerns ought to stop us in our tracks long before we become overwhelmed with the utilitarian appeal of genetic engineering and before the temptation to grasp for control of human life captivates our naïve imaginations.

WHY ENHANCEMENT?

Given that while we might affirm the legitimacy of healing as an aim of gene therapy, we must ask ourselves why we find the aim of enhancement of traits tempting. The question is not even *what* we might like about enhancement, but *why* we like what we like about enhancement. Obviously, there is something appealing in the idea of redesigning one's own physical, emotional, and intellectual makeup. The temptation to do so implies that something is missing in the way we were made by God. Even in a fallen world, in which it is evident that what God intends is not always what is, there is something wrong with our trying to remedy the situation. Remedies are given by God and not everything man is capable of doing is necessarily a remedy, regardless of how it appears to us at the moment.

The moral error in trying to remedy what is wrong with us through genetic enhancement is that we tend to think that enhancement can meet those needs that only God can meet spiritually. The desire for increased bodily strength or skill may be intended, for example, to enhance self-esteem by making us more competitive so that we might rise above others. It is the genetic dream world of a capitalistic, competitive culture to be the best and to come out on top. Contrary to the American dream, however, being the best and coming out on top is not the highest good according to God. Jesus warned his disciples that it is better to be like a child in relationship to God than to argue about who is the greatest.

THE IMAGE OF GOD

True greatness is not found in attempting to be superior to another, but in accepting our being created in the image of God and redeemed through Jesus Christ. "God created man in his own image, in the image of God he created him; male and female he created them" (Genesis 1:27). These words serve as the foundation of our objection to gene therapy for enhancement of traits. It is important to understand what is meant by the image of God. Unfortunately, we often begin our search at the wrong end of the equation. We start with ourselves as human beings and project our human image onto God. It doesn't matter that for some the projection of the human image is a physical one, as if God must then have a body as we do, or whether, for the more sophisticated, the image projected is that of our own desired or actual characteristics or attributes. In each case, the assumption is that the meaning of the image of God begins with us. It does not.

There are some today who define what it means to be human according to the presence or absence of certain characteristics: consciousness, reasoning, self-motivated activity, capacity to communicate, and presence of self-concepts. Accordingly, those who do not display these characteristics are non-humans and are therefore dispensable. Such defining away of humanity is convenient for justifying abortion and euthanasia.

But being created in the image of God has nothing to do with bodily or personal characteristics and attributes. It has everything to do with our *relationship* with God. Martin Luther writes:

> My understanding of the image of God is this: that Adam *had it in his being* [emphasis mine] and that he not only knew God and believed that He was good, but that he also lived in a life that was wholly godly; that is, he was without the fear of death or of any other danger, and was content with God's favor.[1]

To be created in the image of God means to be created in the kind of relationship with God that is shared by no other creature. As Luther says, "The rest of the animals are designated as footprints of God, but man alone is God's image...."[2] The central theme of the Story God tells is one of the loss and recovery of the image of God. The image of God is the perfect relationship with God with which God endowed Adam and Eve. In the beginning before the Fall, Adam and Eve lived in perfect harmony with God because there was no sin and the curse of sin which is death. In the Fall the image of God as this perfect life and relationship with God was lost. Yet, since the

Fall, by God's grace, we are not entirely cut off in our relationship with God. We may be enemies of God, but God loves His enemies. The Gospel of Christ's death and resurrection has brought about the restoration of the image of God for those who have faith in Christ. To put it more accurately, the image of God begins to be restored in this life by grace, through faith in Christ, but it will not be finished in this life. Until we get to heaven, the life we live will not be entirely transformed by the benefits of the Gospel.

THE GOSPEL, GENE THERAPY, IMAGE OF GOD

The Gospel provides what genetic engineering can only claim to provide through the enhancement of traits. It is tempting to think that if we were only smarter or stronger or more skilled, we would then be happier. We look for our fulfillment not in our relationship with God but in our enhancement of the image of man. When we set out to enhance ourselves through redesign of the human genome, we stray farther from the image of God, the faith relationship with God that alone provides what our quest is really about. By identifying, as social scientists do, our physical, emotional, or intellectual characteristics as the sum of all we are that gives us worth, we continue to move away from God as the source of all fulfillment. We futilely attempt to find our worth in our own ability to enhance and control our own potential and destiny.

In spite of the faults and limitations of human nature, the Gospel of Jesus Christ means this:

> So we do not lose heart. Though our outer nature is wasting away, our inner nature is being renewed every day. For this slight momentary affliction is preparing for us an eternal weight of glory beyond all comparison, because we look not to the things that seen but to the things that are unseen; for the things that are seen are transient, but the things that are unseen are eternal. (2 Corinthians 4:16–18)

The Christian's response to the awareness of limited human capabilities is not to trash and redesign the human genome but to make it clear that we are God's creation. More than that, having been justified by Christ, the image of God is restored. We are a new creation, re-created in His image. We inherit the benefits by grace through faith. Geneticists may aim at fulfillment of human potential in genetic makeup, but real fulfillment is found in God's redesigning our relationship with Him through Christ. Our meaning, joy, and peace are found in a good relationship with God. Because of this Paul can write:

> We are afflicted in every way, but not crushed; perplexed, but not driven to despair; persecuted, but not forsaken; struck down, but not destroyed; always carrying in the body the death of Jesus, so that the life of Jesus may also be manifested in our bodies. (2 Corinthians 4:8–10)

That which God has done in Christ and announced as the Gospel is our ethic. It enables us to resist the temptation to determine our own worth and destiny through genetic enhancement of our traits. The Gospel transforms us into far more than genetically superior human beings. It transforms us into the image of God.

HUMAN EMBRYO RESEARCH

The use of human embryos or fetuses for research illustrates the wrongful attitude underlying much of genetic engineering. The understanding of what can be done and what is necessary to do seems to change every day. Among many scientists, the guiding rule seems to be that almost anything science is capable of doing should be done.

Some years ago scientists held out the promise of fetal tissue as the cure for such diseases as Parkinson and diabetes. Time has proven these speculations to be in error. But the attitude which fought to justify trying remains with us today. One ethicist, sympathetic to the use of embryos for research exposed his faulty thinking when he posed the question, "Are human embryos so special that not even lifesaving medical benefits can offset the moral costs?" "Morality" has become expendable. This illustrates the continuing utilitarian nature of the ethics of science. As C. S. Lewis often pointed out, this usually means the death of some for the betterment of others. Under Bill Clinton, in May 1999 the President's National Bioethics Advisory Committee reversed its prior ban on embryo research, saying, "This research is allied with a noble cause, and any taint that might attach from the source of the stem cells diminishes in proportion to the potential good which the research may yield." It is claimed that the end always justifies the means so long as the means supports our aims.

Politics always seems to play a role in genetics. Special interest groups, usually pharmaceutical companies or burgeoning genetic corporations, armed with patent in hand, stand in the wings to enhance, not society's welfare, but their own profit. In January 1999, the Director of the National Institutes of Health demonstrated the technicalities that skirt whatever laws can be put in place to limit genetic research morally. He said that a legal opinion relating to embryo research has now ruled that an organism is only human if it has developed to a live birth human being. This is consistent, of course, with prior legal rulings that denied infants in the womb their humanity if the mother chose to abort her child for any reason. Ethicists not shaped by God's Story tend to reshape their ethics according to the whims, wishes, and trends of the times.

It is not clear as of this writing what new ways and means will be found to manipulate "left-over" embryos or create new ones as "commodities" with which to conduct experiments. There is no law in the land that prevents anyone from doing these activities, and in our fragmented society it seems unlikely we will be able to enact any such legislation. Up until now, laws have only limited funding in an attempt to give society time to evaluate the morality of such endeavors.

Whatever limits are proposed almost always merely cite the "risks at this time" and not the morality of the issue. Christians, however, view such matters in the light of all human life coming from God. Whether developmentally only hours old following fertilization or many years old, all human life is created by God. All human life either bears both the potential for full life on earth as intended by God or is in fact that potential fully realized in old age. According to God's Story, there is no difference in worth between the two. Sin may cut life short through the hubris of geneticists and abortionists or through the plagues and tragedies of a fallen creation. But human beings are held accountable for their destruction of what God has made and will value for all eternity. Those who would tamper with God's creation should think twice, for "it is a fearful thing to fall into the hands of the living God" (Hebrews 10:31).

CLONING

In 1996 the first evidence of successful cloning was presented to the world in a sheep named Dolly, a female clone. Within three years, a male clone was created named Fibro, a male mouse. Dolly was created from an embryo formed when a cell from her udder was inserted into an egg from her own ovary after removing the egg's DNA. Fibro was formed combining a non-reproductive cell clipped from his tail and an egg from a surrogate mouse whose DNA had been removed. The surrogate mouse then carried Fibro to term. At the end of the twentieth century, the number of documented cloned animals (no humans have been cloned) is less than a half dozen in the world. It is not surprising that the possibility of cloning has generally caused negative response from the public at large, positive response on the part of commercial interests, and skepticism mixed with curiosity on the part of the scientific community.

Scientifically, the most fascinating part of cloning is not merely the ability to reproduce asexually, but the possibility of being able to continue life indefinitely through the cloning of body parts that normally wear out with aging. Studies done of Dolly's DNA, however, indicate that Dolly is older genetically than she is chronologically. It appears that DNA ages and a clone made from its own parent cell begins life as a clone, where it left off before cloning, at the same age as its own parent cell. Although this seems to predict a shortened life span for clones, there is great interest in attempting to redesign the substance in a cell called telomere which causes aging. Telomere is a substance at the tip of the cell which, as it divides, also erodes as a cell ages. The assumption is that if telomere can be controlled, clones, whether animal or human, can live forever. Man's dream of immortality continues.

There is much that could be said about human cloning, but human cloning is unnecessary, confusing, and meaningless. There is much that can be said about human cloning, but human cloning is unnecessary, confusing, and meaningless. Do not think the previous sentences a typographical error. I have cloned the first sentence to make a point. This duplication of sentences adds nothing meaningful except to illustrate its own absurdity. In truth, the duplicating of these sentences is unnecessary, confusing, and meaningless, except to reinforce the point. Similarly, human cloning is unnecessary because it adds nothing to our life that God has not already done in the context of our relationship with Him and with one another. Human cloning is confusing because it distorts the truth of the human need to be recreated in the image of God rather than having the image of man presented to us. Human cloning is meaningless because the only ultimate meaning there is comes from God, who meaningfully creates all things new.

Apart from the intriguing possibilities open to man's curious scientific nature, the attitudes and aims of cloning need to be examined from the perspective of the Holy Scriptures, the Word of God. Cloning humans is at least a decade away according to the most liberal scientific predictions. Christians could well delay attempting to seriously determine the implications of cloning according to God's Word, but as with embryo research, the failures of the present scientific endeavors ought not comfort Christians and delay a response on our part.

Christians must respond to the underlying arrogance that takes upon itself the task of redesigning the universe one cell at a time. We must also respond with warning to the search for immortality apart from "putting on immortality" promised us as a gift of God's grace by faith in Jesus Christ. The cross can never be traded for genetic research. As good as many of the results from cloning human organs and body parts may be, it is wrong to violate scriptural truths. Those truths include being created in the image of God, the sharing of the one flesh union of husband and wife, the begetting of children as a gift from God, and the integrity of the body as well as the soul. No "good" that violates these can be justified by what man might call "the betterment of mankind."

It is too soon to know what the age of genetics will bring us, but Christians do well to hesitate, withhold approval, and think critically when media broadcasts announce the latest breakthroughs, and when the "good" resulting from a break-through seems to outweigh the things we are all too quickly willing to sacrifice to obtain them. In the end, the only justifi-cation for much of what is done is utilitarian, and Christians will always remember that having the capacity to do some-thing does not mean we ought to do it. Truth will always out-last the next Tower of Babel created by mankind.

Concluding Thought

Admittedly, this book may not be convincing to non-Christians and, for that matter, perhaps to some Christians. But Christians, as people who live by the Story God tells, ought to look for their ethical guidance in the meaning of what God has done in Christ and not simply accommodate to the world around them. Christians ought not have their ethics defined by the world, nor be overly influenced by it.

In the church, we need not be left merely with ethics based on Law, although there is a place for Law. Sinful human nature needs the Law to show us God's will and our failure to live up to it. If we Christians grasp the meaning of the Gospel for ethics, not as what we do for God but as what God does for us, then there is hope in living ethically and morally by the power of the Holy Spirit within us. The Gospel transforms our lives. As it does so, Christian influence in bioethics will not be limited to trying to find common ground of agreement with non-Christians through the application of Law. Rather, ours will be a witness to the work of God in the holy lives of a holy people.

NOTES

[1] *Luther's Works,* Vol. 1: Lectures on Genesis 1–5, Jaroslav Pelikan, ed. (St. Louis: Concordia Publishing House, 1958), pp. 62–63.

[2] *Ibid.*

Appendix
The Path Of Medical Ethics

The path of medical ethics begins for western civilization with the ancient Greeks, approximately 400 years before the birth of Christ. Preceding and paralleling the Greeks, the earliest Hebrews shared one thing with the ancient world. Both recognized the unity of body and spirit and drew no line of distinction between the practice of medicine and the practice of religion. Hippocrates and Moses were part of the classical view of the world as a unity. This worldview continued until the period in history known as the Enlightenment, usually identified with the eighteenth century. At this time the separation began, in western thinking, between science and faith. Medicine and religion began to pull away from each other.

It was not until the twentieth century, the 1970s in particular, that what had been called "modern medicine" gave way to "postmodern medicine." Modern medicine, beginning with the Enlightenment, was characterized by the authority, objectivity, and duty of the profession of medicine. Postmodern medicine rebelled against these, favoring instead autonomy, subjectivity, and moral relativism. An anti-technology attitude developed with regard to such things as life-support machines, tube feedings, and radical surgeries. The outcome of postmodern medicine has been a rejection of the

Hippocratic Oath and the promotion of abortion, infanticide, physician-assisted suicide, and euthanasia.

At the turn of the millennium however, there seems to be a desire to return to the uniting of medicine and religion. Even psychiatry, previously hostile to religion, has become interested in religion, offering training for psychiatrists in how to teach courses in meditation, miracles, and mindfulness. Much of the interest in spirituality is pagan and mystical, ultimately preaching a religion of self. But the openness of this generation to the uniting of medicine and religion provides opportunity for Christians to speak biblically of the connection, demonstrating the oneness of life in Christ. Medicine and religion united offers the opportunity to restore objective meaning in the practice of caring for patients. It is a door to recovery of the Hippocratic Oath and the Judeo-Christian practice of "Care, if not cure, but do not kill."

CLASSICAL TIMES

ANCIENT TIMES TO THE AGE OF ENLIGHTENMENT

We may identify classical times as that period of history from the time of the ancient Greeks, approximately five hundred years before Christ, lasting until the beginning of the eighteenth century to what has been called the period of the Enlightenment. A pervasive worldview of varying forms characterized the classical period, which differed significantly from what came to be known as modern and postmodern times. The word classical then may refer not only to a period of time, but also to a worldview and a heritage, which is with us today.

One of the chief characteristics of the classical worldview is a belief in the supernatural. This supernatural worldview allowed for a more inclusive view of reality as compared with the later modern worldview in which only the material world was believed to constitute reality. Although the classical world-

THE PATH OF MEDICAL ETHICS

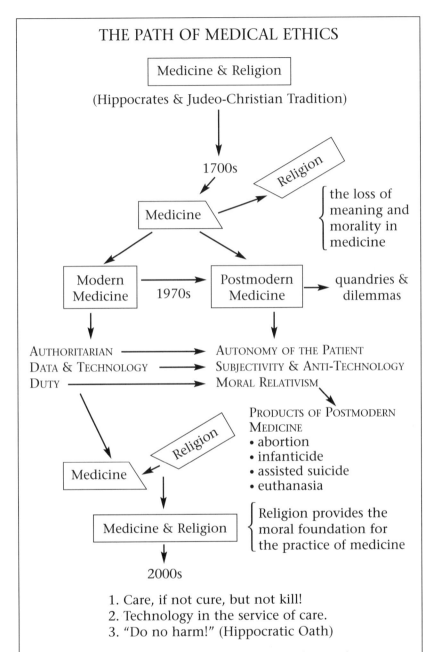

1. Care, if not cure, but not kill!
2. Technology in the service of care.
3. "Do no harm!" (Hippocratic Oath)

The Judeo-Christian tradition gives medicine character, which is moral integrity; identity, as a healing profession; and limits, setting parameters to protect patients.

view was inclusive of a variety of beliefs in the supernatural, the predominant belief that shaped western civilization was the Judeo-Christian tradition. Such a worldview continues to be shared by Christians as a true and accurate description of the larger reality.

Not everything in other worldviews was rejected by Jews and Christians, however. The classical worldview of Jews and Christians did, for example, share some things with the pagan world of the Greeks and Romans. For example, pagans and Christians alike shared a belief in the reality of truth. What they believed about that truth and its accessibility differed greatly, but the ancients did not have to face the postmodern question that claims there is no such thing as truth. The ancient classical pagan worldview shared with Christians the conviction that truth is an absolute, a good conviction on which to build an ethic in any culture.

CLASSICAL ETHICS

Because of a shared belief in common absolutes such as "the good, the true, and the beautiful," ethics from the times of ancient Greece up until modern times was a communal, rather than an individualistic, endeavor. Ethics was founded on a shared commitment to a prescribed behavior expected of those in the community. The ancient *community* of the Greek city-state provided an interpretation of the common good for the good of all. When Greek and Roman civilizations fell, those principles continued to be supported by the Judeo-Christian worldview because many of the moral principles were found to be consistent with the beliefs of Christians. But acceptance of Christian moral principles began to disintegrate during the period of the Enlightenment. These moral principles have all but disappeared as a formative influence in these relativistic and anti-foundational, postmodern times.

Classical ethics may be understood in terms of certain assumptions that characterized its uniqueness. The following statements describe ethics of the classical period:

1. Ethics is about moral development. Ethics is a reflection of the moral character of a person. Ethics is not just what a person does, but what kind of person he is. Accordingly, moral character is formed by practicing virtue. Ethics is a discipline of virtues to be learned and passed on to succeeding generations.

2. Ethics is based on transcendent absolutes. Ethics, as the building of moral character, is based on belief in *absolutes*. Such absolutes exist external to the person, but must be incorporated by the person to become a person of character.

3. Ethics is the identification of the "good, true, and beautiful." Ethics attempts to *identify* or *discover* these qualities. Ethics does not subjectively create them. The essence of ethics is the search for these things.

Moral development, transcendent absolutes, and identification of the good, true, and beautiful are defined by the community of which the person is a part. The life of the community, unified by common belief, defines the moral development of the individual.

MODERN TIMES

EARLY MODERN TIMES: RATIONALISM

Modern times had an early (1700s) and a later (1800s) period. The early period, also called the period of the Enlightenment, was characterized by rationalism (reliance on reason alone to explain reality). The word "Enlightenment" implies that the enlightened person is one who has thrown off belief in the supernatural and relies on reason rather than divine revelation to describe this world. Faith was identified as "superstition" and belief in the supernatural was therefore rejected. This legacy of atheistic rationalism is still with us today in some scientific corners.

During the period of the Enlightenment, the Christian faith was exchanged for the rationalistic religion of Deism. Deism held a rational, anti-supernatural view of God as creator of the world, but one who no longer participated in its daily affairs. Deism was consistent with a worldview in which physical reality was believed to be all that can be known. Reason and science superceded faith.

LATE MODERN TIMES: ROMANTICISM

> C. S. Lewis wrote, "'then came Romanticism and tearful comedy' and the 'return to Nature' and the exaltation of Sentiment; and in their train all that great wallow of emotion which, though often criticized, has lasted ever since."[1]

The late period of modernism was characterized by romanticism. Romanticism was a reaction against the coldness of unfeeling rationalism. It offered a softer, more subjective view of the world. Whereas rationalism relied on reason alone, romanticism appealed to the senses and to personal feelings. Modern romanticism, like earlier rationalism, also rejected the Christian faith, but for different reasons. Romanticism rejected the Christian belief in the limited divine revelation of the Bible claimed by Christians and favored the idea that God is revealed in nature as nature. A romanticist comes to know God by knowing himself since we are all part of nature. Where rationalism rejected the transcendent revelation of the Word of God, romanticism identified spiritual reality with the immanence of nature and the self.

This later modernism is characterized by an abiding faith in science, the self-sufficiency of the individual, and by what, in America, came to be known as Transcendentalism. Those espousing Transcendentalism taught that the solution to human problems lies in the free development of the individual spirit. Transcendentalism, like Deism, rejected the Christian faith, which had claimed an authority outside the self for revelation of truth.

A NEW MORALITY

A new morality emerged under modernism. Since modernism no longer allowed for transcendent absolutes, morality had to be redefined in terms of reason alone, not faith in divine revelation. Applying reason, rationalism allowed for only one foundation for morality, the standard of utilitarianism. Utilitarianism is the belief that the measure of good and evil is the outcome of one's efforts and decisions. In the end, only that which works for me is identified as good and that which doesn't accomplish my goals fails to meet the standard. It was a morality modeled after an emerging, materialistic science, which demanded proofs, as a validation of what is true, and what is not true. The search for truth lost its philosophical and theological origins and became identified with "facts." Eventually the promise of "a better world through science" caused the collapse, for many, of the need for faith in God. The Deism of the Enlightenment gave way to the Pantheism (worship of nature as God) of romanticism. In the end, Atheism (disbelief in God) was born during the modern period.

Later modernism gave birth to the social sciences. The basic needs of man for community and identity, once defined by the Christian faith, were now defined in terms of *social planning* and *psychology*. Social planning aimed at meeting the basic human need of mankind for community. Psychology aimed at helping people live with themselves in their new-found freedom. Unlike the classical worldview in which it was believed that community and identity was to be found in the faith community, the need for community and individual identity in modernism believed these could be fulfilled in the individual's discovery of himself.

POSTMODERN TIMES

FROM THE 1960s TO THE PRESENT

Modernism gradually developed into postmodernism because the promises of rationalism and science failed to deliver, and in fact, created new problems. Postmodernism rejected the authority of reason. Today, in postmodern times, people no longer seek an objective rational foundation for ethics, but instead seek personal subjective meaning in pursuit of their own morality. At the same time, even as transcendent absolutes are rejected, postmodernism also rejects any materialism that excludes the possibility of the supernatural. Spirituality is defined as each man's personal, subjective search for meaning within himself based on his own feelings and experiences of the world around him. Postmodernism rejects the rational atheism of modernism and offers instead a spirituality that makes a religion of anything and everything one subjectively believes to be true.

The dominant philosophy of postmodern times is existentialism. Although Kierkegaard, the father of Existentialism, emphasized personal choice only as way of authenticating faith, his emphasis deteriorates under postmodernism into choice for choice sake. By the middle of the twentieth century, the notion of "choice" included the choice to reject tradition and authority altogether.

EXISTENTIALISM TODAY

The chief characteristic of the philosophy of existentialism is belief in the self rather than in abstract universal ideas. One method of fostering existentialism is through *values clarification* which calls for the individual to form his own opinions about truth rather than accept what others have handed down to him. Kierkegaard said truth is real for us only as it becomes personal, but he personally did believe in truth as revealed in the Word of God, the Bible.

As a rebellion against established ideas and institutions constructed on abstract ideas, existentialism today opposes the Judeo-Christian tradition, which gave rise to those ideas and institutions. Existentialism as a philosophy is in opposition to Christian dogma (teachings), but existentialism as an influence on all our lives shapes even those within the Christian Church. For example, the emphasis on personal conviction, always present in the Christian faith, now in the environment of existentialism, has become more authoritative than Scripture itself. Existentialism believes that truth (being subjective rather than objective) is whatever I make it to be. According to existentialists, each person finds truth for himself in his own experiences of life. Ethical discussions are, consequently, a matter of shared *opinions* rather than about classical truths uncovered over the centuries.

Pragmatism, another name for utilitarianism, is the basis for interpreting life experiences. For example, in ethics committees in hospitals the search is not for universal truth, but for *pragmatic solutions.* The ethics of health care today is not interested in morality or in the meaning of the choices we make, but concerns itself only with practical problem solving on the part of each autonomous person, each man or woman finding what is right for him or her. This stands in contrast to a Christian understanding of truth as given by God and affirmed by faith. The human will, not the will of God, becomes the authority behind ethical decision-making.

In these postmodern times we have lost the deeper meaning of life and we feel the frustration evident in our preoccupation with power. Power always turns to violence as it does when abortion, infanticide, and euthanasia are proposed. Modernism had tried to bring order and structure to life rationally and scientifically. Postmodernism encourages the opposite. It encourages *chaos*, which is the result of unrestrained freedom of choice. Postmodernism does not build. It deconstructs, dismantles, and tears down. Any attempt to absolutize answers through rational or spiritual means is rejected.

Postmodern times could be described as a move from the atheism of modernism to the nihilism of postmodernism. Nihilism is the conviction that nothing matters. We must create our own *virtual reality*. Nihilism knows no moral or ethical limits. Christians have opportunity in postmodern times to offer authentic Christian teachings that help people find truth. There is a mystery to life that can only be fully known spiritually as God reveals it. What we have talked about as classical turns out, in part, also to be eternal and good for all times, especially relevant in postmodern times which has lost all solid foundation for living.

SITUATION ETHICS

"Only one thing is intrinsically good;
namely, love: nothing else at all."[2]

Joseph Fletcher also wrote in 1966, "Situation ethics goes part of the way with natural law, by accepting reason as the instrument of moral judgment, while rejecting the notion that the good is 'given' in the nature of things, objectively. It [situation ethics] goes part of the way with Scriptural law by accepting revelation as the source of the norm while rejecting all 'revealed' norms or laws but the one command to love God in the neighbor. The situationist follows a moral law or violates it according to love's need."[3]

LOVE MAKES RIGHT

Situation ethics, as articulated by former theologian Joseph Fletcher, attempts to avoid two extremes. It seeks, on the one hand, to avoid an ethic based on absolute rules that cannot be bent, and on the other, to avoid an ethic that rejects rules altogether. Fletcher insisted that there is one rule and one rule only that is valid, the *rule of love*. He claims to find this rule of love in the New Testament, but believes this love to be *relative* rather than *absolute*. When faced with a dilemma which cannot be resolved without violating a moral principle, that moral principle can be set aside in the name of love, for love determines what is moral. Fletcher's rule of love then becomes the justification for violating all other rules and prohibitions. If, for example, the rule is that a person should not lie, "for the situationist what makes the lie right is its loving purpose. If a lie is told unlovingly it is wrong, evil; if it is told in love it is good, right."[4] Fletcher's view stands in contrast to Christian teaching, as articulated by Gilbert Meilaender, that we are not to do all the good we can, but only all the good we can morally do."

THE LESSER OF TWO EVILS

Luther recognized that people in real life situations are often faced with a choice between two evils. He urged the Christian to choose what in a biblically enlightened conscience he believed to be the lesser of the two evils and to "sin boldly," believing more boldly in the mercy of God which forgives our sins. Luther did not intend by this that it doesn't matter whether you sin or not, but was attempting to point out that in a fallen world all choices are tainted by sin. We must choose, at times, among the lesser of these, genuinely repent and trust in Christ. Fletcher believes there is no need for repentance or forgiveness since doing the loving thing makes evil good. Fletcher has no concept of sinful human nature, which affects our motives and actions. The obvious weakness in Fletcher's view historically is that people in the name of love have performed terrible atrocities. In love, a father shoots and kills his entire family because he doesn't want them to have to face the kind of world in which we live. A mother destroys her infant child because the court is about to take her child away from her. As Gilbert Meilaender says, there are limits to what God allows us to do even in the name of love.

Although Fletcher's situation ethics claims to make "love" the deciding factor, the real principle at work is utilitarianism. Love, according to Fletcher, always serves a purpose! Love is always a means to an end. The resolution of a dilemma is the aim of love.

In situation ethics dilemmas are resolved on a case by case basis. Because there are no absolute principles to follow, each case is isolated from every other case. There are no preconceived notions of right or wrong. This case by case method of approach to ethics is also called casuistry. In casuistry, each case needs be resolved, not by moral rules, but by the good intentions of well-meaning people. Situation ethics are not concerned with moral theory but with offering good reasons why we ought to do one thing rather than another. Situation ethics assumes that each person knows all he needs to know about himself, the situation, and the outcome he intends.

THE THEORY OF PRINCIPLISM

In *Principles of Biomedical Ethics,* published in 1989, Tom L. Beauchamp and James F. Childress proposed an ethic based on principles, the idea that universal principles can govern ethical decision-making in medical ethics. They write, "In defending a rule-governed concept of morality, we have implicitly rejected situation ethics."[5] "However, we will now argue that the model of absoluteness for moral rules is the wrong model."[6] They go on to suggest that rules are binding, but not absolutely binding. These rules govern not so much morality as they do the procedures most of which are aimed at protecting patient's rights.

In principlism there is a shift in ethics from teaching morality, to guaranteeing the patient freedom from external moral influence by others. It is said, over against a classical model of ethics, that "ethical theory does not create the morality that guides professionals decisions and actions."[7] Therefore, discussion no longer focuses on determining what is moral, but on what procedural matters will guarantee the patient the right to determine subjectively what is moral for him. Principlism is primarily a utilitarian approach to ethics, justified on the subjective basis of each person's emotive response to suffering and the prospect of death.

Principlism does not claim to have a foundation on which to base moral judgments. Beauchamp and Childress admit that what we decide morally depends on what we believe [religiously] about the world, but they do not explore the relationship between morality and principles. They do say, "… controversy about human life and personhood is impossible to decide on the basis of the moral principles that form the core of principles in this book."[8] This means, in effect, that morality is left to each person to decide for himself. In a postmodern world this usually means utilitarianism and emotivism.

Principlism, as proposed by Beauchamp and Childress hinges on the principle of autonomy. Autonomy is not so much a principle for ethics as it is a defense against outside influence that seeks to bring moral meaning into ethical debate. In all, these authors propose four principles but autonomy dominates the other three and becomes their interpretive guide.

These four principles are:

THE PRINCIPLE OF AUTONOMY

"The principle of respect for autonomy does not determine what a person ought to be free to know or do or what is to count as a valid justification for restraining autonomy."[9] The principle of autonomy seeks to protect the patient from undue influence by guaranteeing the right to privacy and the right of informed consent before treatment. Ultimately, the only limiting factor in the exercise of one's autonomy is that one may not do harm to others in the exercise of his own autonomy.

THE PRINCIPLE OF NON-MALEFICENCE

This principle aims at preventing harm to a patient. It allows, however, for what is called "double effect" harm, meaning that harm may result although it was not intended. Measuring harm is based on such criteria as "quality of life" and the "patient's best interests." The principle of autonomy is an overriding influence on implementation of this principle.

THE PRINCIPLE OF BENEFICENCE

There is an attempt to balance the principle of non-maleficence by the principle of beneficence. Not only ought we avoid harm, but we also ought to *help* the patient. *Help* implies acting out of mercy or compassion. Although this principle is well-intended, in the change of direction in medicine from "healing" to "the relief of suffering," the aim of helping the patient may now suggest help through physician-assisted suicide or euthanasia.

THE PRINCIPLE OF JUSTICE

The basis of this principle is that patients ought to be treated fairly. This means equal access to health care and proper allocation of resources. Again, although well-intended this often deteriorates into less medical care for the weakest and sickest in order to reduce the costs of health care. In a postmodern, utilitarian culture, economics plays the lead role in national discussions of health care. Money can be saved by not treating people.

These principles serve as general or universal guides to action. The problem with principle-based ethics is that there is no foundation on which to base an interpretation for implementing these principles. Principlism turns out to be antifoundational in its subjectivity. For example, these principles could be used to both provide or deny medical treatment and reject or promote the killing of patients. Since autonomy plays a major role in quandary ethics there can be no shared community to help us interpret these principles.

"The 'principlist' method seeks to fashion a minimal morality for a community of strangers, even if friendly strangers. A bioethics fashioned for this purpose will offer a lowest common denominator agreement."[10] And it will omit dealing with matters on which people disagree such as the nature of being human, the meaning of suffering, etc. It tends to serve as a basis for creating public policy, but does little for personal moral guidance and personal moral integrity.

QUANDARY ETHICS

The approach to medical ethics concerned with following ethical procedures, rather than with what is understood traditionally as moral values, is called Quandary Ethics. Quandary Ethics focuses on the quandary or question raised by the situation and seeks to determine what to do, rather than what is moral. "What to do" focuses on utilitarian or emotive concerns rather than on questions of right and wrong. The inherent nature of quandary ethics is to avoid moral judgments and seek practical solutions based on the principle of autonomy.

ASSUMPTIONS

Quandary Ethics makes certain basic assumption that ethics is about solving problems.

Ethics is about choices. The focus of Quandary Ethics is not on the moral development of the person or even on what the person believes about life, religiously or otherwise. In Quandary Ethics the person as person is not part of the decision he makes. The assumption is that the kind of person I am has little or nothing to do with what I do. This can be seen in today's political climate where the immoral lifestyle of a President of the United States seems to have little or no influence on citizens' beliefs about whether he can do the business of politics well or not. This same divorce between and a man and his behavior can be seen in the media portrayal of Jack Kevorkian as a good person under attack by the authority of the courts. Although once a doctor, sworn to heal patients, Kevorkian kills patients and moral outrage against what he does has been slow in coming. It is as if it can be said of Kevorkian, "Just because he kills people doesn't mean he is a bad person." The assumption of contemporary ethics is that the action we take can be separated from the kind of person we are.

Ethics is about moral values as neutral. We have come to believe of ourselves that, accurately or inaccurately, as a society there are so many different thoughts about morality that we cannot hope to find any common moral ground in medical ethics today. One way to deal with diversity of moral values is to declare all moral values and the choices that derive from them equal. If all values are equal then all choices in bioethics are value-neutral choices. Quandary Ethics builds on the idea that there is no absolute moral foundation. Quandary Ethics is, in fact, anti-foundational, and challenges anyone who claims to have an exclusive claim on Truth. Christian morality is particularly under attack since it claims exclusive truth and has been the foundation of our moral thinking for two millennia. Quandary Ethics seeks to deconstruct Christian moral influence on ethics.

Ethics is about following principles. Principlism aims not at moral development but at solving medical dilemmas or answering medical quandaries. Although principlism does not propose a moral principle of its own as does situation ethics in proposing love as the guiding principle, principlism does propose general subjective principles such as autonomy, do no harm, do good, and justice for ethical decision-making.

Quandary Ethics is virtually the exclusive way of thinking about ethics in health care today. This approach affects thinking in everything from abortion to euthanasia and yet Quandary Ethics as an approach to ethics has failed. Merely identifying quandaries and providing procedures to enable people to make their own decisions on the basis of personal values is, in reality, abandonment of the patient who is asking for answers about what to do. We are faced with more questions than answers and biotechnology continues to present more quandaries every day. Something more than method is needed, something like content that is biblical and true for all time.

The AMA Code of Ethics

The American Medical Association was founded in 1847. In part, it appears to have been founded on self-interest as the articles of incorporation say, "for the protection of their interests, for the maintenance of their honor and respectability, for the advancement of their knowledge, and the extension of their usefulness" (*JAMA*, Oct 8, 1982, Vol. 248, No. 14). The motivation for its formation in large part was the exclusion of "quacks" referring to homeopathic doctors and apothecaries.

The Code of Ethics of the AMA has undergone many revisions since the days of its founding, changing already in 1903 and more recently in 1996. An editorial in the *Journal of the American Medical Association (JAMA)* August 5, 1996 reports, "The AMA's Code of Ethics today is a constantly evolving document that serves as a contract between physicians and their patients. Responding to current trends, the code is developing new boundaries for the *business* of medicine" [emphasis mine]. This editorial comment in *JAMA* raises some red flags regarding the purpose of a code of ethics.

First, that the standard for moral behavior with reference to the Code of Ethics should change according to "current trends" makes one wonder whether doctors are expected to abide by the Code or whether the Code is to be adapted to the practices of doctors. If the Code is a standard to live by it seems a strange matter to revise the Code to conform to the behavior that is obviously beyond the prior limits set by the Code. The same editorial elaborates, "the ethics which govern it [AMA] must keep pace with progress." How interesting that the changes in moral behavior in medicine *should* change and that such change is necessarily seen as "progress."

Second, it will not come as any surprise to many that the word "business" has replaced the word "profession" in reference to medicine. What is a surprise is that the medical establishment should unashamedly use the word. Perhaps it is for this reason and the political nature of the AMA that membership is declining among young doctors who have a better view of medicine and their profession. In spite of this decline in membership and the fact that the AMA represents close to half the doctors in America, the Courts nevertheless continue to recognize the AMA as representative of physicians in America in making judgments on ethical questions in medicine.

Ethicist Arthur Caplan writes that it was in 1980 that the first significant revision of the Code appeared identifying the new *principles of medical ethics* that exceeded the norms that ought to be followed by physicians in private practice "into the much more murky ethical waters." But perhaps the AMA cannot be faulted any more than we can fault our society or those trends within it which tend to relativize ethics and violate traditional standards of all kinds. The Code of Ethics of the AMA is merely a reflection of life in these postmodern times. As Christians we ought surely to be a light in the darkness of medical ethics today. The void left in the world by the fall of ancient Rome was filled by Christians who introduced truth to the world in the person of Jesus Christ.

THE IMAGE OF GOD
AND THE HUMAN GENOME PROJECT

Having been created in the image of God, means that Adam and Eve were created righteous. Being created in the image of God does not have so much to do with having similar characteristics man shares with God, but rather has more to do with the nature of the relationship man has with God. No other creature created by God is described as having this kind of relationship. One ethicist, trying to reconcile biblical meanings with ethical dilemmas proposes that being made in the image of God means having certain traits that make us human, such as self-awareness, consciousness, intentionality, etc. The implication for this ethicist is that if any of these traits are missing in a debilitated person they no longer qualify for being human and therefore created in the image of God. The outcome is that we may dispatch such persons in response to the ethical dilemma facing us.

But being made in the image of God is not about the quality of life, it is about the quality of the relationship we have with God. Before the Fall human nature was good and in harmony with God. That relationship cannot change with deterioration of physical or mental status. The relationship we have with God is constant because God is constant. But the relationship has changed since the Fall because human nature is now sinful from the moment of conception. Since the Fall, no human being possesses the perfect relationship with God, described as being made in the image of God, except God who became man, Jesus. We find that restored image in our being made by God's grace in Jesus Christ and His suffering, death and resurrection for our salvation. This gift is ours through a faith relationship with Jesus Christ in which the Holy Spirit works love for and trust in God in us.

But even with the loss of the image of God in those not restored to God in Christ, the idea of the image of God is still a valid criteria for measuring God's intent for what it means to be a human being. Those in whom the image of God is restored by Christ know God's intent for all people and therefore can evaluate proposed ethical solutions on the basis of their faith relationship with God in Christ. The redeemed, by virtue of their faith relationship, can distinguish truth from error when ethical proposals are measured over against the written Word of God. They can, for example, evaluate the proposals that emerge from the findings of the Human Genome Project, which has mapped out the function of each human gene, to determine whether they are compatible with the Christian faith or not. Christians can begin by asking what are the implications for being made in the image of God in reference to the Human Genome Project?

Some distinctive observations can be made. First, although being made in the image of God is not a physical or mental image, we know from the Word of God that God highly values our bodily existence. We dare not de-value it due to injury, illness, or birth defect, but ought to honor and respect all human life regardless of human evaluations of quality of life.

Second, even though the image of God was lost in the Fall, and in some it will never be restored due to absence of faith in Christ, we still know God's desire is to restore the image in all. Because this is so, we must value every person as one potentially to be restored by God. God is still at work in all of us by grace working to repair the damaged done and to restore every person to the image of God.

Third, we must be careful not to define what it means to be human by the capacity of genetic makeup, human intellect, emotion responsiveness, social interaction, or other human criteria. To be human and to be a person worth every bit as much as any other is to be made in the image of God. In the beginning, God set that aim in motion and carried it to fulfillment in His Son, Jesus Christ our Lord.

Fourth, since the Human Genome Project, which looks to some version of the story of evolution as its foundation and makes no distinction between man and animal, makes no provision for spiritual meanings, we ought to be careful not to allow genes to define us, refine us, or redesign us. It would be sin to begin to think that human life could be given fulfillment by merely remaking us genetically in the image of the new man, where we value for the moment what we believe to be important for a full life.

Attempting to reconcile our being made in the image of God with the findings of the Human Genome Project will lead us to perform atrocities that future generations will suffer. Man's destiny is not to be determined by attempts to focus on genetic makeup, thereby excluding the less tangible, spiritual relationship which sets moral limits to human endeavor. It may not be a violation of the Word of God to seek gene therapy for purposes of curing disease, and yet it may become a violation because we are sinful human beings, capable of atrocity and error. But it is surely morally wrong for us to attempt to re-design the human genome for purely aesthetic or enhance-ment purposes because these are not the things that give life worth or meaning. As such, they take attention off what God has made us to be spiritually. Such attempts at enhancement or redesigning of the human genome are, at the core, attempts to avoid the only meaning God gives, which is that we are crea-tures created by a Creator. We are not our own masters and our lives are not to do with as we please.

Notes

[1] *The Business of Heaven,* Daily Readings from C. S. Lewis, 1984, p. 157.

[2] Joseph Fletcher, *Situation Ethics* (Philadelphia: Westminster Press, 1966), p. 57.

[3] *Ibid.,* p. 26.

[4] *Ibid.,* p. 65.

[5] *Principles of Biomedical Ethics* (Beauchamp & Childress, 1989), p. 47.

[6] *Ibid.,* p. 51.

[7] *Ibid.,* p. 394.

[8] *Ibid.,* p. 162.

[9] *Ibid.,* p. 72.

[10] Meilaender, *Body, Soul, and Bioethics* (Notre Dame: University of Notre Dame, 1995), p. 18.

Bibliography

Beauchamp, Tom L., ed., *Intending Death: The Ethics of Assisted Suicide and Euthanasia* (Upper Saddle River, NJ: Prentice Hall, 1996).

Beauchamp, Tom L., and Robert M. Veatch, *Ethical Issues in Death and Dying*, 2nd ed. (Upper Saddle River, NJ: Prentice Hall, 1996).

Beckwith, Francis J., *Politically Correct Death: Answering Arguments for Abortion Rights* (Grand Rapids, MI: Baker, 1993).

Bork, Robert H., "Inconvenient Lives," *First Things* 68 (1996): 9–13.

Bottom, J., "Facing Up to Infanticide," *First Things* 60 (1996): 41–44.

———, "Christians and Postmodern," *First Things* 40 (1994): 28–32.

Cameron, Nigel M. deS., *Life and Death after Hippocrates: The New Medicine* (Wheaton, IL: Crossway, 1991).

Kilner, John F., Nigel M. deS. Cameron, and David L. Schiedermayer, eds., *Bioethics and the Future of Medicine: A Christian Appraisal* (Grand Rapids, MI: Eerdmans, 1995).

Cole-Turner, Ronald, *The New Genesis: Theology and the Genetic Revolution* (Louisville: Westminster/John Knox, 1993).

Drlica, Karl A., *Doubled-Edge Sword: The Promises and Risks of the Genetic Revolution* (Reading, MA: Helix Books, 1994).

Feinberg, John S. and Paul D. Feinberg, *Ethics for a Brave New World* (Wheaton, IL: Crossway, 1993).

Fletcher, Joseph, *Situation Ethics* (Philadelphia: Westminster Press, 1966).

———, *The Ethics of Genetic Control* (Buffalo: Prometheus, 1988).

Fuchs, Josef, *Personal Responsibility: Christian Morality* (Washington DC: Georgetown University Press, 1983).

Kevles, Daniel J., *In the Name of Eugenics: Genetics and the Issues of Human Heredity* (Cambridge, MA: Harvard University Press, 1985).

Pope John Paul II, *The Gospel of Life Washington, DC: United States Catholic Conference, Evangelium Vitae.* March 25, 1995.

Hauerwas, Stanley, *Community of Character* (Notre Dame: University of Notre Dame Press, 1981).

———, *Suffering Presence* (Notre Dame: University of Notre Dame Press, 1986).

———, *Naming the Silences* (Grand Rapids, MI: Eerdmans, 1990).

———, *After Christendom?* (Nashville: Abingdon, 1991).

Hauerwas, Stanley and Alasdaire MacIntyre, eds., *Revisions: Changing Perspectives in Moral Philosophy* (Notre Dame: University of Notre Dame Press, 1983).

Hilton, Bruce, *First Do No Harm: Wrestling with the New Medicine's Life and Death Dilemmas* (Nashville: Abingdon, 1991).

Hughes, William E., "The People versus Martin Heidegger" *First Things* 38 (1993): 34–38.

Jansen, Waldemar, *Old Testament Ethics: A Paradigmatic Approach* (Louisville: Westminster/John Knox, 1994).

Kaiser, Jr., Walter C., *Toward Old Testament Ethics* (Grand Rapids, MI: Zondervan, 1983).

Kass, Leon R., *Toward a More Natural Science: Biology and Human Affairs* (New York: The Free Press, 1985).

———, "What's Your Name?" *First Things* 57 (1995): 14–35.

Kilner, John F., *Life on the Line* (Grand Rapids, MI: Eerdmans, 1992).

Kreeft, Peter, *Making Sense Out of Suffering* (Ann Arbor: Servant Books, 1986).

Lammers, Stephen E. and Allen Verhey, eds., *On Moral Medicine: Theological Perspectives in Medical Ethics* (Grand Rapids, MI: Eerdmans, 1987).

Lee, Patrick, *Abortion and Unborn Human Life* (Washington DC: Catholic University of America, 1996).

Lejeune, Jerome, *The Concentration Can* (San Francisco: Ignatius, 1992).

Lifton, Robert J., *The Nazi Doctors* (New York: Basic Books, 1986).

MacIntyre, Alasdair, *A Short History of Ethics* (New York: Macmillan, 1966).

———, *After Virtue* (Notre Dame: University of Notre Dame Press, 1981).

Mappes, Thomas A. and David D. Grazia, *Biomedical Ethics*, 4th ed. (New York: McGraw-Hill, 1996).

May, William F., *Active Euthanasia and Health Care Reform* (Grand Rapids, MI: Eerdmans, 1996).

Meilaender, Gilbert, *The Limits of Love* (University Park: University of Pennsylvania Press, 1987).

———, *Faith and Faithfulness* (Notre Dame: University of Notre Dame Press, 1991).

———, *Bioethics; A Primer for Christians* (Grand Rapids, MI: Eerdmans, 1996).

———, *Body, Soul, and Bioethics* (Notre Dame: University of Notre Dame Press, 1995).

———, "Begetting and Cloning," *First Things* 74 (1997): 41–43.

———, "Second Thoughts about Body Parts," *First Things* 62 (1996): 32–37.

———, "The Eclipse of Fatherhood," *First Things* 54 (1995): 38–42.

Mitchell, Basil, *Morality: Religious and Secular* (Oxford: Oxford University Press, 1980).

Nelson, Paul, *Narrative and Morality* (University Park: Pennsylvania State Press, 1987).

Olasky, Marvin, *Abortion Rights: A Social History of Abortion In America* (Washington DC: Regnery, 1992).

Pellegrino, Edmund D. and David C. Thomasma, *The Virtues in Medical Practice* (Oxford: Oxford University Press, 1993).

Russo, Enzo and David Cove, *Genetic Engineering* (Oxford: W. H. Freeman, 1995).

Schulz, Gregory, *The Problem of Suffering* (Milwaukee: Northwestern, 1996).

Smedes, Lewis B., *Choices: Making Right Decisions in a Complex World* (San Francisco: Harper, 1986).

Veatch, Robert M., *Medical Ethics*, 2nd ed. (Sudbury, MA: Jones and Bartlett, 1997).

Veith, Gene Edward, *Postmodern Times* (Wheaton, IL: Crossway, 1994).

Verhey, Allen V. and Stephen E. Lammers, eds., *Theological Voices in Medical Ethics* (Grand Rapids, MI: Eerdmans, 1993).

Walther, C. F. W., *Law and Gospel* (St. Louis, MO: Concordia Publishing House, 1981).